THE
NATURAL
FACE-LIFT

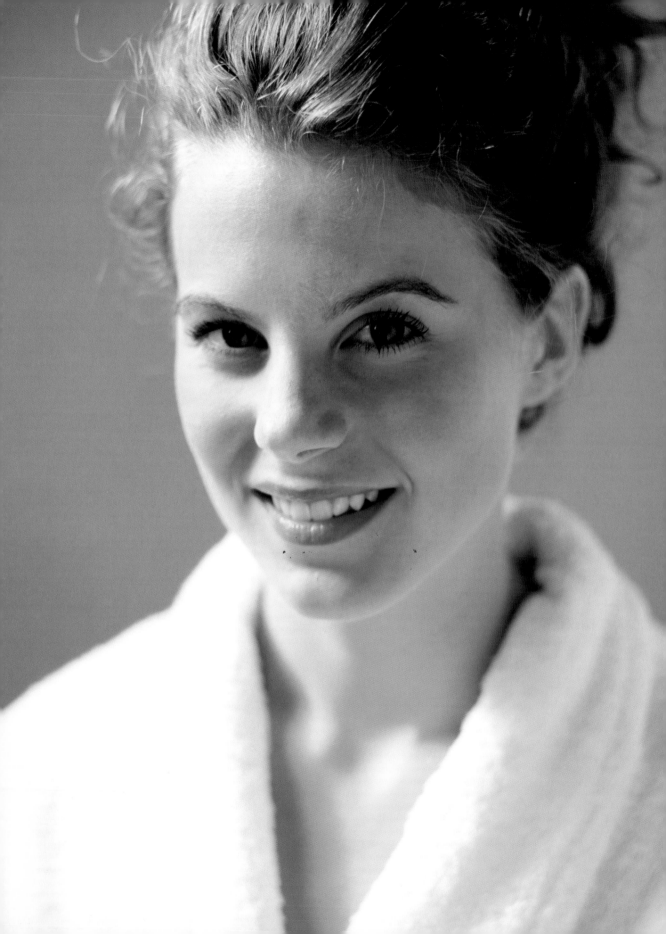

THE NATURAL FACE-LIFT

FACE-LIFT

A Facial Touch Program for Rejuvenating Your Body and Spirit

LINDA BURNHAM, N.D.

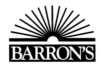

BARRON'S

First edition for North America published in 2004
by Barron's Educational Series, Inc.

First published in Great Britain in 2003
by GODSFIELD PRESS LTD,
Laurel House, Station Approach,
Alresford, Hampshire SO24 9JH, U.K.
www.godsfieldpress.com

Project Editor: SARAH DOUGHTY
Designer: JANE LANAWAY
Photography: MIKE HEMSLEY AT WALTER GARDINER
Photography Models: DAVID CORDELL, MIMI RAOUF,
NICOLA SMITH, ELIZABETH GUNN

Designed and produced for Godsfield Press by
THE BRIDGEWATER BOOK COMPANY

All inquiries should be addressed to:
Barron's Educational Series, Inc.
250 Wireless Boulevard
Hauppauge, New York 11788
http://www.barronseduc.com

International Standard Book Number 0-7641-2629-6

Library of Congress Catalog Card Number 2003100372

Printed and bound in China

987654321

AUTHOR ACKNOWLEDGMENTS

In gratitude: To the Supreme Being who orchestrated this entire project from its inception to its conclusion. To my inner and outer teachers for your constant love and support through all my transformations. To my mother, Gladys Noyd Miller; she taught me about inner beauty and gentle ways to support it—from facial soaks and carrot juice to slant boards and evening meditation. To all my students and my Burnham Systems Facial Rejuvenation Practitioners for hanging in there (some of you) for more than thirty years of transmission and hands-on practice. To Judy Sheer for thinking of me as the perfect author for this book. To Brenda Rosen for understanding my ideas and ushering them into a proposal that worked. To Godsfield Press and Barron's Educational Series, Inc. for taking the leap of faith with me. To Diana Lanier for stabilizing me in body, mind, and spirit through the writing process and the crises of multiple surgeries, hospitalizations, and tedious recovery of a fractured leg. To the staff at the Bridgewater Book Company for their calm acceptance of unavoidable delays due to my accident. To Dawna Page for patiently handholding me through the editorial process into the wee hours of the morning. And finally to Susana (Susie) Castro Leite for literally and figuratively helping me to take each step along the way with humor: synthesizing thousands of pages of transcription into a few hundred words; interpreting the Rejuv experience into a simple text; and translating the complexity and precision of the professional Facial Rejuv work into a user-friendly, self-help protocol. Without her constant assistance on all levels, this book would have remained just another great idea.

CONTENTS

INTRODUCTION

DO YOU EVER WATCH A MOVIE OR LEAF THROUGH A MAGAZINE AND SEE A SPECIAL LOOK AND WANT IT FOR YOURSELF? THE GLOSSY HAIR, SMOOTH COMPLEXION, BRIGHT EYES, AND PERFECT SHAPE OF A MOVIE STAR OR MODEL ARE DEFINITELY ALLURING. YEARNING FOR THE BEAUTY OF A PARTICULAR STYLE OR ERA IS NOT UNUSUAL. MANY OF US DREAM OF ACHIEVING SUCH BEAUTY. IS THAT BEAUTY REAL? IS IT INSTEAD SIMPLY THE SKILL OF MAKEUP ARTISTS, HAIRSTYLISTS, LIGHTING DIRECTORS, AND A GIFTED CAMERA CREW?

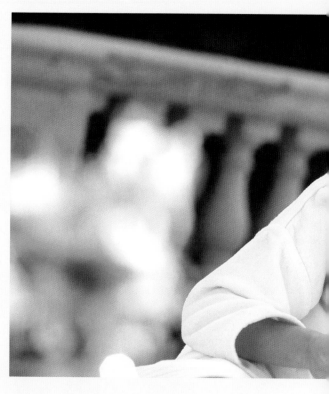

Style is often considered what is in vogue. Style makes a statement, but ultimately an ephemeral one, subject to change with each season and advertising campaign.

The Natural Face-Lift is about taking our relationship to beauty beyond the external markers of transient style and glamour. Books on beauty often focus on the face, addressing the skin topically and therefore remaining on the surface of the issue. This book will take you deeper, to the true seed of your unique beauty.

This seed contains all the possible responses to whatever life may offer—the good, the bad, and the ugly. Vital and compelling beauty is the radiance sprung forth from this seed. It is a unique radiance, your personal frequency of light and color. You generate it and offer it to the world with every interaction. Although we have a wide

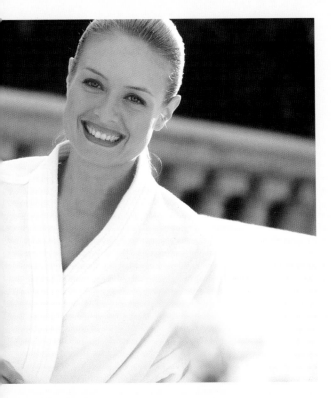

infirmity, uselessness, and decay. However, this attitude is limited and erroneous. In truth, aging is the accumulation of life experience growing into wisdom. When our values are in harmony with our thoughts and actions and we have distilled a sense of peace from our laughter and tears, the aging process can become a precious part of life.

Each of us carries within us a jewel—original and priceless, a composite of the genetic, karmic, familial, and cultural facets that makes us unique. We are rarely told about this inner treasure, much less shown how to nurture and polish this jewel into a dense, brilliant, multifaceted gem—the reflection of our true essence. We are born into this three-dimensional world to work and play within a vast arena of possibilities. We move through life either reacting or responding. This book is about understanding how life experiences translate into the stories faces tell and how recognition of trauma and release can help us rewrite them.

The Natural Face-Lift is based on the revolutionary techniques of Burnham Systems Facial Rejuvenation—the Rejuv Touch— a unique system of patterned sweeps and touch sequences that sculpts the face and neck and activates major nerve centers. By applying these sequences, you will touch your face with tenderness, replenishing your skin's vitality, nurturing your body, and revitalizing your spirit. The Rejuv Touch routines and rituals for beauty and healing will make your whole body come alive. You will enter a deep state of relaxation. Contractions in facial muscles will be eased. Skin cells will be fed. Nerve pathways will be opened. You will experience a body-wide free flow of vital energy. Your stamina and inner beauty will be revitalized. You will meet the world with a radiant face, a refreshed body, and a renewed spirit. The Rejuv Touch has the potential to change your life by awakening the beauty beneath your skin.

range of mental abilities and the full spectrum of emotions to respond to the gifts and challenges of our daily lives, we often limit ourselves to a small and restrictive range of responses, in particular, "It's just who I am." The range we choose will determine our habitual patterns of response and set our musculature into lines of expression.

This book is not just about experiencing a natural face-lift. It is also about maximizing the vitality of your body, renewing your spirit, and enhancing your zest for life. The Natural Face-Lift is not about reversing the signs of aging. Mass marketing and demographic targeting have convinced us that in order to enjoy real quality of life, we must be youthful. The by-product of this indoctrination is that many of us now feel uncomfortable about growing older. We see the visible signs of aging and often equate them with

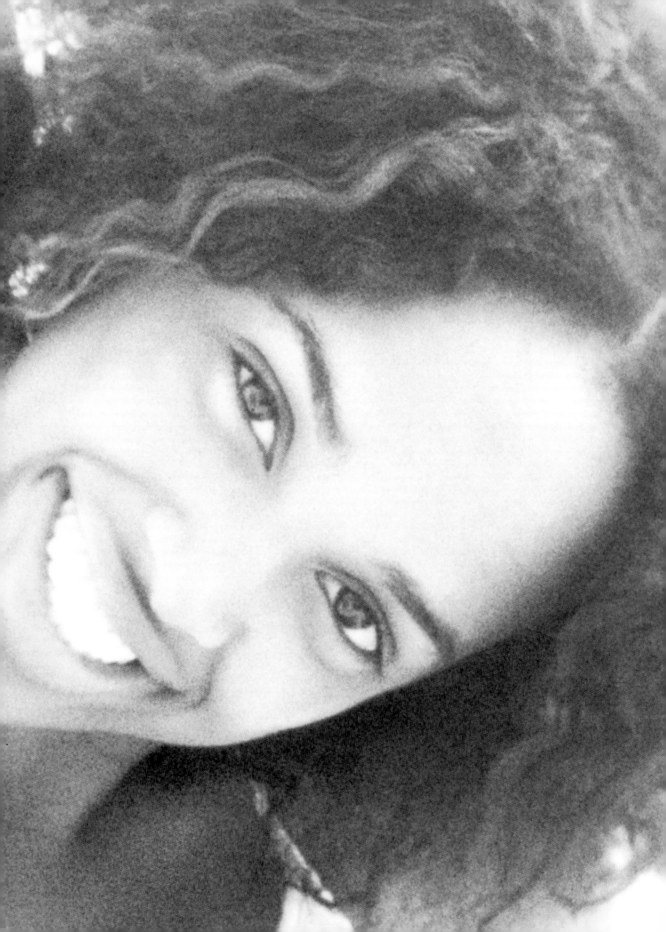

PART ONE:

THE ART OF BURNHAM SYSTEMS FACIAL REJUVENATION

Each of us responds differently to life. We react to situations based on genetics, history, fears, vulnerabilities, dreams, and strengths. Our individual responses and reactions impact all our levels of being—physical, energetic, emotional, mental, and spiritual. With tenderness and consciousness of the body's innate wisdom, Rejuv approaches the depths of our being. We explore how trauma is registered and released, and how nourishment on each level of our being defines our quality of life, physical vitality, and the face we show the world.

The concepts in Part One are distilled from Dr. Linda Burnham's model of physical-spiritual medicine. Its multidimensional approach to health, beauty, and healing makes Burnham Systems Facial Rejuvenation both practical and transformational. These physical–spiritual concepts are embedded in several thought systems (physical sciences and quantum physics, practical spirituality and mystical traditions, natural herbal and nutritional guidelines). They are based in deep reverence for the extraordinary wonder of the human body and psyche.

The art of the Rejuv Touch is to free the matrix of traumatic experiences, release trapped energy, and enliven the bony structures and facial musculature, thus reflexively allowing the natural alignment of body, beauty, and spirit.

1. OUR FACES, OUR STORIES

YOUR FACE IS YOUR CALLING CARD. IT IS THE FIRST IMAGE OF YOU THAT PEOPLE RECOGNIZE, AND YOU CANNOT HIDE THE INFORMATION THAT APPEARS THERE. HOWEVER, YOUR FACE TELLS IT ALL— THE COMPLETE STORY OF YOUR LIFE. WE CAN ALL SEE MOODS AND ATTITUDES DANCE ACROSS THE FACES OF FAMILY, FRIENDS, AND PASSING STRANGERS.

The movements of our bodies display our thoughts and emotions through body language. When we would rather not participate, we drag our feet. Our shoulders slump when the weight of our experience seems too much to bear. A furrowed brow may signal an attempt to understand or concentrate during a stressful moment. All of these nonverbal messages can be seen and interpreted by others. Psychologists have shown that 93 percent of communication between human beings takes place through body language while only 7 percent is expressed with words. Although the words themselves may be misunderstood, a scowl or a smile can reveal the true intention.

The face is a region of highly concentrated and integrated body language. The road map of a person's life is impressed into the skin by the mobility of the musculature beneath it. The curves, the lines, and the muscle patterns provide a visual display of the integration of our experiences. Every thought and emotion, every experience at every level of our being, impacts the body and can be read most clearly on the face.

When a particular emotional response runs through us time and again, it activates the same muscles and micromuscles as it did the first time. Disappointment or hurt feelings, for instance, might cause the same narrowed eyes, pursed lips, or clenched teeth each time we feel disappointed or hurt. When a response becomes habitual, the face may "freeze" into a permanent expression. One example of this tendency can be seen in the worry lines that crease the forehead of a perpetually nervous person.

Spend a few minutes looking carefully at your reflection in the bathroom mirror. What curveballs or silver spoons has life offered you that are revealed by the expressions you see in the mirror? How you welcome the gifts and meet the challenges that life offers creates your face—the face that greets the world, the face you cannot hide. If you are not happy with what you see, if lines of strain and sadness are your calling card, the techniques you will learn in this book can help you rediscover the radiant face that expresses your true beauty from beneath the surface of your skin.

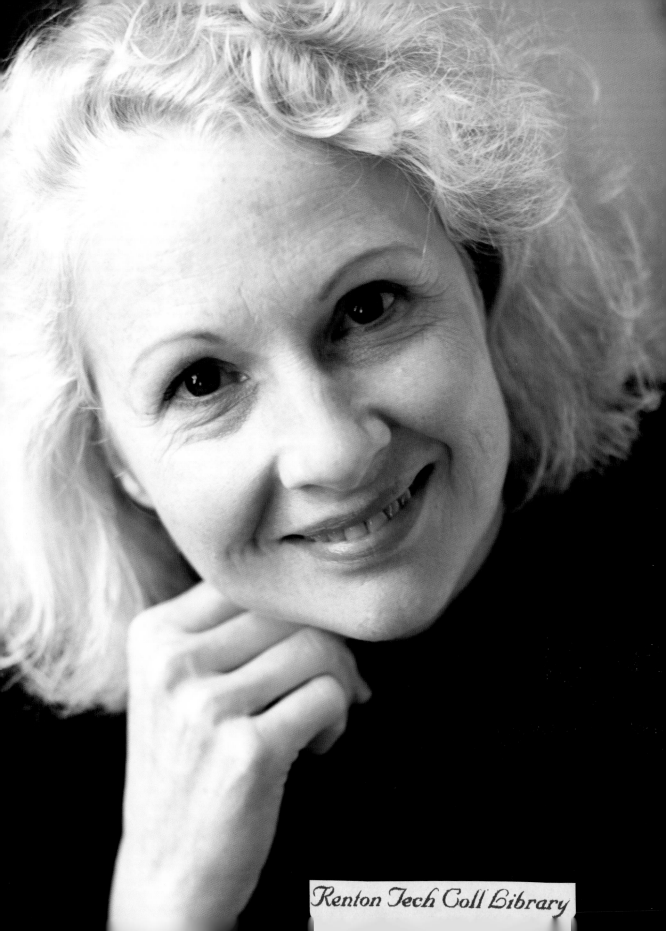

DIFFERENT BUT THE SAME

Each of us is unique; no two people are exactly the same. We are each endowed

with genetic characteristics, cultural and familial idiosyncrasies, learned behaviors,

and individual perspectives. Even siblings describe completely different experiences

of growing up in the same household. Even so, we all have the same basic structures.

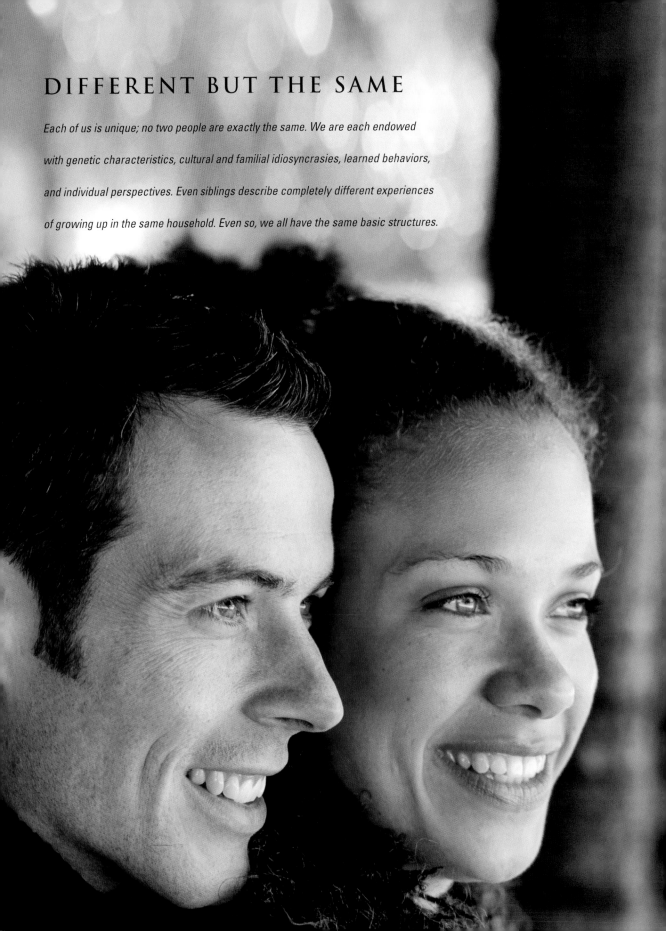

First and foremost, we live in physical bodies. For the most part, though, we all have legs and feet to move us forward, hands and arms to hold and create, and senses that help us understand and take in our world. A complex system of internal organs sustains and regulates life. The multifaceted brain keeps it all going, functioning even without conscious participation.

Within the physical body are energetic structures. The Western medical model is just beginning to embrace this aspect of human physiology. In Eastern medicine, the energy body is comprised of a complex grid of meridians that crisscross the body, within and between the major energetic organs (chakras). Health in this system is the result of an unimpeded flow of energy. The physical and energetic bodies are interwoven with one other; the well-being and health of one profoundly affects the other.

As human beings, we are feeling beings. We feel our world and our lives profoundly. Our feelings seem to rush through our body, so we grasp at them, attach them to a story line, label and store them as emotions. Later, we can access the memory and tell the story in all the glorious or gory details of the experience.

When we access our memory banks, we employ conscious thought. The story becomes fixed with information and evidence supporting a particular point of view. Our thoughts and opinions seem so solid—almost immovable. However, physically they are just a compilation of chemical and electrical responses within the cerebral cortex. Although our brains receive, sort, and store an avalanche of sensory data on a daily basis, our thoughts are what make sense of our world.

Beyond these four bodies—physical, energetic, emotional, and mental—is the still, small voice of spirit. Called by many names, this essence animates the flesh, fulfills the emotions, and calms the mind. This ultimate source of all life ignites life itself within each one of us. When your spiritual self has completed its time on this planet, your personal sojourn is also over.

Each of these five bodies penetrates, or permeates, all the other bodies within the physical body. Each bodily aspect is separate. However, they are all interconnected and woven together to create each unique human being. Our focus in this book is to discover and use simple ways to bring ourselves back into our natural alignment.

TRAUMAS

Our life purpose is as varied as our personal philosophy. However, all of us have experienced the highs and lows of existence. The highs lift us and open us to more of what life has to offer. The lows tend to bring us down, contract us to the next moment. The ability to function as a whole, complete being is hampered by a contraction in any area. By contraction we mean a trauma to the system. Low moments are often recorded in the body as traumas.

Traumas—mental, emotional, or physical—can be large or small, meaningful or insignificant, remembered or forgotten. The structures of our energetic and physical bodies retain the memories. Some traumas impact us profoundly yet we can release them almost instantly. Other traumas are carried deep in the psyche and musculature and may be released only years later.

When we experience trauma, the communication and balance between the energetic and physical bodies is compromised. The two bodies begin to separate, just slightly, at a cellular level—the physical and energetic bodies go out of phase with one another. This slight separation results in a loss of their ability to nourish and sustain one another. We become more prone to the forces of gravity—we sink, we drop, we collapse, we age. What seems like a natural progression could be an unnatural consequence of the stress of unreleased traumas at the cellular level.

Contractions can occur on any level, even in the densest part of the body—the bones. Although bones seem hard and brittle, they are living tissue undergoing constant regeneration. We will focus our attention on a connection between the bones of our hands and the bones of our faces to release contractions on any level. Bones support us in every way—giving structure and form to our bodies and helping us stay upright within the force of gravity as we move forward.

When we think of the law of gravity, we may vaguely recall some scientific information about the nature of the planet. Simply put, gravity causes Earth to orbit around the Sun, people to stay on the ground, and objects to have weight. From the time we are conceived, we are affected by gravity. As babies, we explore and experiment with this force. We drop items from great heights: food from the high chair, toys from the crib. These repetitive actions may annoy our caregivers. In tangible ways, though, they allow us to experience the scientific information that Newton quantified. As we grow, we learn to move our bodies from crawling to standing and finally to walking upright, an awesome evolutionary moment. The physical aspect of any sport would be impossible without gravity. We can only dance, jump, and run because of this universal force. That is the good news.

The trouble begins when we stop playing with this force and become unaware of its effect on us. Our bodies begin to collapse, and we begin to age from the constant downward pull. A prolapse (dropping or lowering) can happen to any part of our anatomy. Different areas of our skin begin to sag and bag: jowls, necks, upper arms, and even bottoms. Our faces show the same signs in eyes, lips, and chins. All of these little sags are prolapses. They signify that part of the cellular integrity has been lost and the ability of physical structures to stay toned and upright in response to gravity has diminished. Superficial prolapses can be embarrassing or annoying, but prolapse of the internal organs can even be life threatening.

Our physical bodies respond to the gravity of the planet, while our emotional and mental bodies respond to the gravity of life. Whether or not our life situations are difficult, we can allow our thoughts and emotions to make them challenging. Whether the moment was truly painful or a negative attitude made the situation less bearable, the emotional response creates a strong, dense impact on the physical body. When we take a heavy view of what life has offered us, or when our emotional and mental attitudes are somber, the effect of gravity is even stronger on our bodies. At these times, we are more likely to collapse into ourselves. We sink in response to the situation. The weight of gravity, coupled with a bleak outlook, can cause our bodies to show even more stress and strain.

Despite the challenges and traumas we may experience, we are hardwired to withstand all that life has to offer us. The toddler who is learning to walk has an infinite capacity to fall and yet never give up in the face of adversity—gravity. Her resilience is based in the harmony or alignment of our mental and physical bodies.

Over time, the physical force of gravity, the seriousness of our emotional and psychological outlook, and our negative behavioral patterns drag us down. All of the traumas of our lives, whether we remember them or not, are held and remembered in the body. The contractions of our muscles and bones, especially those portrayed on our faces, ultimately reveal our life stories.

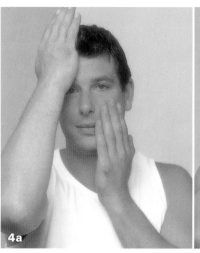
4a

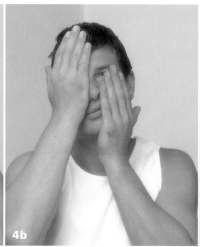
4b

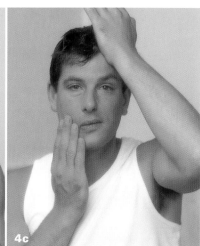
4c

THE GRAVITY EXPERIMENT

This simple exercise illustrates how the downward pull of physical gravity affects the musculature of your face. During this exercise, notice not only what happens to your face but also what happens to your energy, your thoughts, and your feelings. The most important principles of the Rejuv work—expanding, opening, and uplifting—take on a new significance when we contrast them with the force of gravity.

1. Take a close look at your face. Notice your features—not only your physical features but also the quality and tone of your skin and the energy emanating from your face (about 2 inches [5 cm] from the skin's surface).

2. Rub your hands together until you feel warmth between them.

3. Warm the skin of your face with both hands. Notice how you feel.

4 a–c. With firm strokes, simultaneously use one hand to sweep up, from the chin to the forehead, and the other to sweep down, from the forehead to the chin.

5. Sense the texture of the downward drag over one side of your face.

6. Examine your face again, observing the energy in front of your face and considering your feelings about what you see.

7. Look and feel for as long as you like, then repeat step 3.

8 a–c. Slide both hands from chin to forehead and off the top of your head.

9. Examine your face, your energy, and your feelings once more.

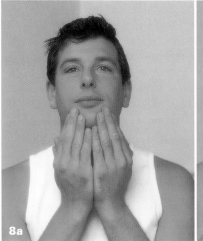
8a

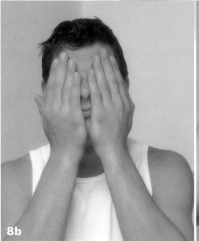
8b

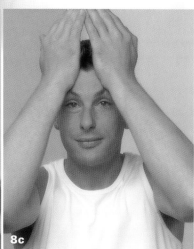
8c

Even simple events—a ringing phone that startles us, being asked to meet a tight deadline, stubbing our toe—can produce momentary muscular contractions. These tiny contractions, although not specifically traumatic, affect the cellular and energetic fabric of our being. The moment of contraction, usually indexed to the emotional content of the situation, creates a tiny knot. We call this knot an *emotional crystallization*. Regardless of the level in which the contraction was triggered, both the energetic and physical levels will move slightly out of alignment.

This minute contraction may be registered in the cells of a cheek, a kidney, or deep in the colon. Somewhere, something has gone awry. When a few cells are out of phase, we usually do not register it consciously but the body remembers. Despite these little shocks, we usually bounce back and continue our activities. However, with repeated minor traumas, the physical tendency is to continue going awry in the same area.

The body holds different types of impacts in different areas—such as, fear in the kidneys, anger in the liver, grief in the lungs. Major traumas cause us to contract even more intensely. When these experiences, situations, or interactions are labeled as negative, we register anger, fear, or anxiety and add to the number of emotional crystallizations within the body. This is how our personal stories are developed: Our emotions or our bodies get hurt. We nurse our wounds, we stop flowing with the moment, and we get stuck. Not only are thoughts and emotions stuck in the experience, but the experience itself is stuck in the physical and energetic crystallizations.

Over time, we may begin experiencing physical symptoms such as saggy jowls, a prolapsed colon, or a nagging pain. Our original intentions were not to create disease but to protect ourselves from uncomfortable situations. Facial expressions are a clear indication of how we have integrated what we have experienced. Bringing more of our selves into wholeness requires dissolution of these emotional crystallizations. Our feelings (before they were labeled and we attached our story line to them) were free-flowing life force, moving through our sensory systems as nourishing energy—the juice of life—for our use on all levels. We can alter the stories written on our faces not by denying the painful experiences but by releasing the emotional crystallizations with a gentle touch.

Our intention is to reweave the energetic and physical bodies together into greater wholeness. We use the Rejuv Touch to soften and loosen the emotional crystallizations. This process does not require us to relive the situation or to experience a dramatic emotional release. Focused intention and attention simply allow the contracted energy to dissolve and reenter the system. We use the nerve centers and pathways of the head to work the entire body reflexively. As the emotional crystallizations dissolve, the physical and energetic systems realign and the life force can flow freely through the area again. When we bring our selves back into harmony, we can experience life more fully.

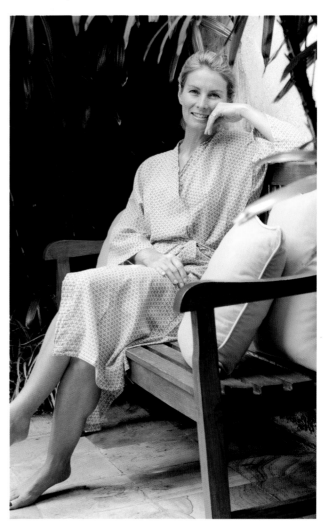

WRINKLES

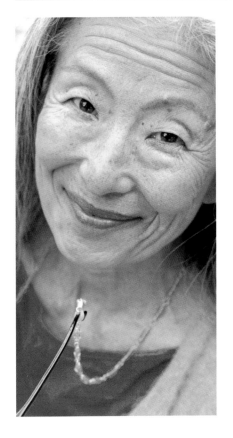

Aging is an inevitable process of life on this planet. How we age and where we show or feel our age, though, are unique to each of us. The most noticeable effects of aging are found in the flexibility of the skeletal system, the tone and elasticity of major muscle groups, and the condition of the skin, particularly the complexion. Many factors come into play in the individual aging process—genetics is the baseline, followed by emotional and mental responses to life circumstances; dietary choices, including the use of caffeine, alcohol, or tobacco; the level of pollution in the environment; and the amount of exposure to Sun and wind, to name the most significant. A given combination of these factors either replenishes or drains our regenerative abilities and our physiological responses and also determines the depth of the lines set in our faces.

Thousands of times in a single day, we use our facial muscles to communicate, thereby slowly creating lines of expression—crows' feet around the eyes, laugh lines around the mouth, creases across the forehead. Lines of expression reveal each individual's unique character. They display our inner reality as our muscles respond to feelings and thoughts. However, these lines can become permanent wrinkles when the micromuscles contract in response to unresolved emotional situations. In this contracted state, blood flow to the tissues is limited—nutrition and hydration are unable to reach the cells and the metabolic elimination is slowed. Over time, the tissue around the contracted musculature is damaged, not only from the lack of circulation but also from the emotional crystallization. The crystallized emotional pattern, locked into the multiple levels of being, is expressed by the wrinkle.

CELLULAR COMMUNICATION

The Rejuv Touch is quite different from other facial work because of its focused contact with major cellular communication. When we contract on any level—energetic, mental, or spiritual—our physical musculature conforms by also tightening and contracting. By using inner or verbal communication while touching and energizing major nerve centers and pathways, the potential for release of contractions and rejuvenation is greater. Nothing is magical or complicated about this process; we know the body responds to thoughts and emotions. We possess the ability to encourage our cells to let go and relax.

Cellular communication affects the biological, biochemical, and bioelectrical responses. We can remind every cell in every bit of tissue to relax stress and tension, let go of old holding patterns, and release past wounds and judgments. This communication will enliven the entire area. The micromuscles begin to relax, and the physiological structure of the area begins to change. By using the Rejuv rituals, we can literally release the physical ties that bind and open ourselves to receiving deeper energetic flows into every area of our lives.

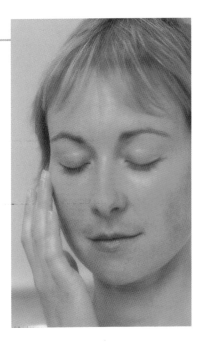

Life's Little Traumas—A Story

When Mary was born, her parents were delighted to have a little girl join them and their three-year-old son, Johnny. Life was grand. Mary and Johnny became pals and did everything together. When Mary was three, Johnny started kindergarten. Mary looked forward to her big brother coming home from school each day.

Johnny was having new and interesting experiences at school. He learned to play hide-and-seek with a new twist. When he least expected it, someone would jump out of the hiding place and yell, "Boo!" This was scary at first, but great fun to hear the other kids scream, then laugh. It was a good joke.

In order to share this new game with Mary, Johnny decided to hide around a corner and jump out when Mary walked by. Mary not only screamed but also cried and ran to Mommy. Her beloved brother continued to scare her at least once a week. She always screamed and then cried. After a while, Mary knew it was Johnny, but she still got scared every time. She learned to walk around corners very cautiously. By the time she herself started school, however, all had been forgotten.

As a teenager, she often had the strange feeling that if she could not see around a corner, it was not safe to proceed. Offered a chance for a Junior year abroad, at first Mary looked forward to the opportunity, then she reconsidered. She did not connect this feeling with Johnny's game. She was not being paranoid; she simply had an unconscious emotional crystallization at the root of her uneasiness. The course of her life changed because of the subtle contraction of an unintentional childhood trauma.

Mary has since grown up. Unconsciously, she still braces herself before turning a corner, afraid of the unexpected. She lets opportunities pass her by. She is somewhat nervous about loving people, and she feels a need to be prepared for what someone may do to her. For years, she carries her cautious thoughts, "I have got to watch these corners because I do not know what is going to come out at me. I cannot move without looking; I know it is not safe" as the best way to take care of herself.

This example of the energetic matrix created from a simple childhood experience is not devastating, but the trauma is far-reaching. We all have traumatic moments. Large or small, they are stored in some level of our being. As other moments add to the area of contraction, we become stuck and build habitual patterns of response—physically (a permanent scowl, tight lips, hunched shoulders), energetically (erratic, flighty, manic), emotionally (victim, bully, caretaker), or mentally (stubborn, indecisive, inflexible). These emotional crystallizations are manifested in our musculature, in our organ systems, in our auric field. All are connected like a giant jigsaw puzzle—all fitted together—different pieces, different parts.

On the journey of life, healing is possible. Someday, Mary can decide, "I'm tired of being afraid. Something is holding me back and I don't want to live with it anymore." Like her, you may find yourself saying, "There's got to be something more. I feel so constrained, what's the next step?" Quite simply, the next step is to relax. Relaxation is a gateway to release. When you are relaxed, you can trust enough to release. When you release, you let go. When you let go and surrender to your inner being, to your needs, to your own flow, you are allowing the source of life to realign you with your true radiance.

You can take these steps toward release with a friend, a therapist, a trainer, a workshop, prayer support, or even a good book. Even with a small step, you may notice that part of a crystallization is released. It may still be there, but it is a little lighter to carry. Follow your heart, your intuition, the still, small voice leading you to release the old ways and participate in new events with an open mind. You may need years to release the patterns of a lifetime, but one day you will realize that you have changed.

The changes will happen, bit by bit, layer by layer. No matter how many layers of crystallization or trauma are bound, healing is available and on some level, we all want to heal. As we long to be whole and free, we embark on the rare and precious journey of our own healing; yet, we are not on it alone. When we share our stories, choose to release judgments and hold ourselves and each other in love—even for an instant—in that instant, crystallizations are released. Traumas are released, and one day the very last one just goes; it has gone, and from that moment on, we are free. That is the nature of multidimensional healing. It is healing on all levels; it is transformational.

The Rejuv Touch is based on a simple premise—touching one area of the body affects the whole being. It is not just a physical reflexology system; it is a way to integrate all the bodies back to their original wholeness. You can spend a lifetime processing and healing all your emotional situations so that the body, weighed down by the gravity of those situations, can begin to let go. Alternatively, you can spend a few moments daily, fully present with yourself, lifting off all the excess baggage with the touch that transforms.

In the Rejuv Touch process, we use our hands to bring our bones into a new balance. By redefining the bony structure, we refine what makes us beautiful and what makes each of us unique. As we energize the bones, the muscles are also toned and rearranged into a more natural position. This phenomenon brings a sense of peace and beauty to the face since the muscles are no longer being pulled in many different directions from countless past energies. The muscles will instead rest gently on the bones. This refinement will be visible on your face, in your eyes, in your lips, and even in the way you carry yourself. We access the physical structures of our faces to open, expand, and uplift ourselves. Thus our true radiance is expressed naturally. Using our hands to help reveal our radiance means so much more when we focus on wholeness.

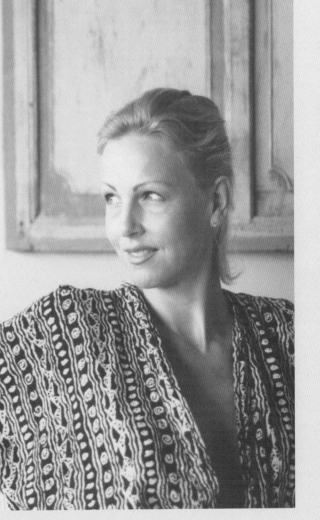

2. THE DETOX KEY

THE BODY IS AN EXQUISITE MECHANISM CAPABLE OF REGENERATION AND REJUVENATION IF GIVEN THE RIGHT RAW MATERIALS. HEALTH AND ITS APPARENT RADIANCE THROUGHOUT THE WHOLE BODY—ESPECIALLY THE FACE—IS A RESULT OF THE INNER WORKINGS OF THE BODY.

What we see on the outside reflects what is happening on the inside. Therefore, proper nourishment is the key to detoxification, purification, and regeneration. A simple statement, and to which we can all agree its validity, but one that is often difficult to put into a daily practice. Our economy may thrive with the convenience of fast foods and bulk buying that seems to support the fast-paced frenzy of our daily life, but the real cost is paid by our health when we suffer increasing amounts of disease in our culture. Our physical problems develop over time. Rejuvenating nutrition allows the body to detoxify and then renew itself on both cellular and systemic levels. Providing the highest quality nutrients to the cells allows them to restore, rebuild, and regenerate all the tissues, organs, and systems of the body to achieve maximum health and vitality.

The Rejuv approach to skin care strives to make it possible for every body system to function optimally. Rejuvenating nutrition, sufficient hydration (both internal and external), and loving touch allow the skin to function efficiently on both mechanical and biochemical levels. Natural, organic, and biodynamic ingredients are presented in a good-better-best approach to detoxification of the internal organs that are ultimately responsible for the condition of the complexion.

Each of us must decide how to nourish the body as well as the heart, mind, and spirit. We want to nourish all aspects of ourselves with the best sources of energy. The choices we make daily, in a consistent manner over time, will determine the quality of our lives. How we prioritize and fulfill the needs of our whole being is the key to vitalizing health and wellness.

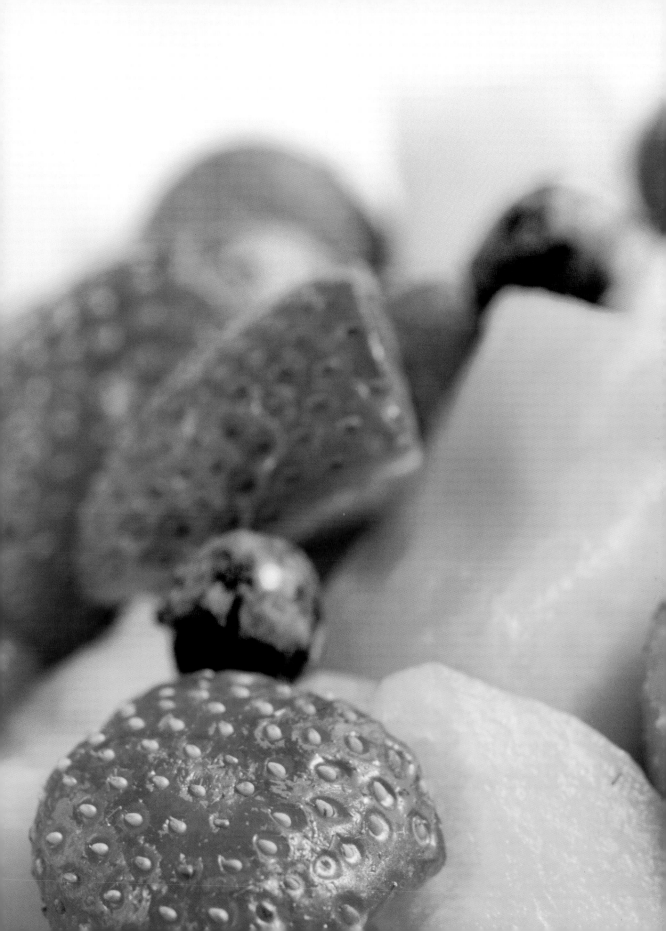

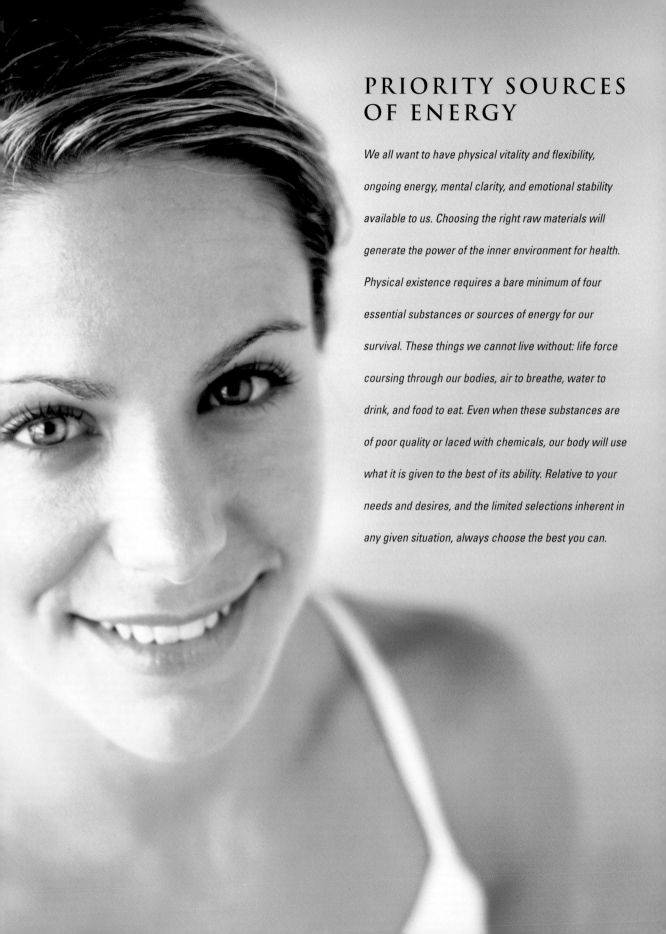

PRIORITY SOURCES OF ENERGY

We all want to have physical vitality and flexibility, ongoing energy, mental clarity, and emotional stability available to us. Choosing the right raw materials will generate the power of the inner environment for health. Physical existence requires a bare minimum of four essential substances or sources of energy for our survival. These things we cannot live without: life force coursing through our bodies, air to breathe, water to drink, and food to eat. Even when these substances are of poor quality or laced with chemicals, our body will use what it is given to the best of its ability. Relative to your needs and desires, and the limited selections inherent in any given situation, always choose the best you can.

Enhancing vitality on all levels becomes possible with conscious attention to these four priority sources of energy. Their order of priority is based on how long we can live without each one: Life force—without this energy we would die immediately. Air—without breath we cannot exist for more than four minutes. Water—many people are in a state of subliminal dehydration, but complete dehydration causes death within weeks. Food—without some nourishment we can survive perhaps a month at best.

We nourish ourselves with these four sources of energy, not merely to survive but to determine a baseline for life. To create a balanced and fulfilling quality of life we also need to rest and exercise, experience love and respect, enjoy purposeful activity, and spend time with family and friends. The quality of these essential substances and how we provide ourselves with them is often a matter of personal choice, habit, and education. Much of our time is focused on the food we place in our mouths. However, we need to pay equal attention to how we feed our senses, our emotions, our minds, and our spirits—the books we read, movies we see, music we listen to, conversations we share, people we befriend, thoughts and daydreams we create. Be sure that these foods have the vitality of the life force in them and they will nourish body, mind, and soul simultaneously.

First Priority: Life Force

Whatever we call this life force—God, divinity, light, divine love, goddess, great spirit, holy spirit, creator—it is our spiritual sustenance. This force is a substance that permeates all creation. It is the cohesive force that binds atoms from the vastness of empty space to create the variety of life-forms as we know them. It inspires our creativity and fuels the desires of our heart. We need to acknowledge and connect with this force in ways that suit our lifestyles and our temperaments. Organized religion, spiritual groups, prayer and meditation, silence, music, nature—find the approach that is right for you. Spend time daily tapping into this source of energy.

Second Priority: Air

Each cell of the body needs oxygen to perform basic metabolic functions. Air contains 21 percent oxygen. The respiratory system is designed to filter from the air toxic chemicals and pollutants, microscopic organisms, bacteria, viruses, dust, and gaseous substances. As we inhale this particle-dense air, our lungs absorb what we need and exhale unnecessary substances and metabolic waste as carbon dioxide. Polluted air in cities or conditioned air in buildings may have the right mix of gases, but they lack *prana*, the Eastern term for the highly charged essence of life. Air near bodies of water and greenery (gardens, parks, forests) is alive with prana. If you cannot be in an environment with naturally living air, then see, feel, and imagine prana surrounding you as golden sparkles of light. Consciously breathe in prana every day.

Third Priority: Water

The simplest, most common compound—water—is the basis of all life on the planet. It is the primary component of our bodily transport systems—saliva, blood, lymph, and urine—as well as the fluid base of all our cells. As such, it absorbs nutrients from one area and delivers them to another. Hungry cells absorb the nutrition and release metabolic wastes to be transported into the organs of elimination. This crucial fluid must be replenished every day for the healthy functioning of not only our physical but also our energetic, emotional, mental, and spiritual bodies. The average adult needs 2 cups (16 oz or 500 ml) of water daily to maintain *each* of the following systems at a minimum: saliva for the mouth and esophagus; moisture for digestion, respiration, and the skin; lubrication for cells, joints, and organs; flexibility for bones; and fluidity for the electrical currents of the nerves. Health is strained when the body suffers subliminal dehydration.

Fourth Priority: Food

Starvation on a cellular level can take a long time. A great many people survive on very poor nutrition. Without any nutrition, though, the body will begin to shut down systems within a few weeks. Across the globe, nutrition takes many different forms, yet the wide range of cuisines will always include proteins, carbohydrates, vegetables, fruits, and oils. Our industrial society has removed us from the fruits of the land and water and instead provided canned and frozen foods that add to our convenience but detract from our health. The body has a limited amount of space to store the chemicals it cannot process. Over time, it will develop unhealthy symptoms from this toxic overload.

The old adage, "you are what you eat," is true. When we feed ourselves life-giving vital foods, we will experience vitality in body and mind. Choosing better raw materials gives the body more to work with; it will regenerate and repair itself more swiftly. Choosing the best nourishment gives the body the best building blocks to vitalize our health and well-being. You can apply the good-better-best rule to anything you choose. Simply be aware and understand your own body's nutritional needs and how to meet them, learn what foods heal and what foods hurt. Then make your choices with ease and confidence.

The choices we have in a modern diet are staggering not only in quantity but in loss of quality through industrial processing and mass marketing. As unique beings with individual preferences and needs, we must familiarize ourselves with the basic principles of rejuvenating nutrition. Human bodies require nutrients from all the food groups. Simply stated, proteins, nuts, and seeds are builders; vegetables are healers; fruits are cleansers; carbohydrates are energizers; and fats and oils are lubricators. Each is necessary for optimal bodily function.

Every human being is born with an enzymatic bank account. An abundant but limited number of enzymes is produced, stored, and used daily. Every metabolic and digestive function requires enzymes. Regeneration takes place on a cellular level as the body withdraws enzymes to repair itself. Vital foods contain enzymes that support the body to break down their nutrients, bypassing the enzymatic bank account. Vital foods are grown in nutrient-rich soil, absorbing life force from the Sun, the rain, and the natural cycle of seasons. This food contains both life force and nutrients that feed every cell of our body.

Devitalized, refined, and processed foods deplete our enzymatic bank account because their nutrition has been compromised. Foods become devitalized when they are grown in depleted soil laced with pesticides. Often harvested early then sprayed with preservatives and waxes, these crops have fewer nutrients and have absorbed all these toxic chemicals. Further processing and refining destroys their enzymatic action. These foods require withdrawals from the enzymatic bank account just to extract minimal nutrition and neutralize the toxins.

The best produce looks like it did while it was still growing. The further from the tree, the greater the loss of nutrition is a

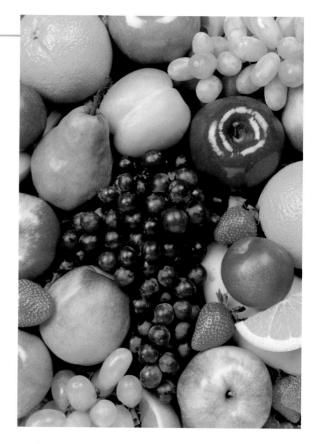

good general guideline to determining high-quality produce. Fresh and raw are better than frozen; frozen is better than canned. Preservatives, pesticides, and genetically engineered produce may all contribute to the visual appeal of the food, but not to its nutrition. The better choice is organic produce, grown naturally to support the crop, the planet, and all people. The best alternative is biodynamic produce, where the soil, the crop, the farm, and the farmer join in the cosmic dance of the natural growing cycle. Remember, the good-better-best rule is relative to the situation. Buy the best you can and energize it (see Chapter 5, "Elixir of Life") to return life force to the food itself.

Rejuvenating nutrition focuses on the quality of the foods we eat and we need to consider what we drink. Our choices today run the gamut from fine wines and gourmet coffee to diet sodas and sugared fruit drinks. Yet our bodies need only pure water! Water—the amazing substance that cleanses, purifies, nourishes, and refreshes everything it touches—is the only liquid we need. Water carries the flow of life force through our body. Whenever you think of getting a drink, reach for water first.

The principles of rejuvenating nutrition support all the organs, systems, and metabolic functions within the body. With cellular and systemic functions taking place efficiently, your skin, eyes, hair, and nails—the naked parts, exposed to the world—will exhibit the radiance, gloss, and resilience of your inner beauty in outer manifestation. To summarize:

Increase water intake from the minimum 8 glasses per day to 12 per day.

Since you do not have the option of not breathing, drinking more water is the first choice toward improving your health. Remember, you are composed of 70 percent water. Therefore, inner and outer hydration are crucial to your health and beauty. Hydration of your face is one of the most important factors in softening the lines and wrinkles that life may bring. Water gently assists natural exfoliation without stressing or damaging the skin. The water in and around each cell needs constant rehydration, not just superficial creams and lotions.

Eat organic and/or biodynamic foods, and use organic/biodynamic products daily.

Because the skin responds to the raw material ingested by the body, the best way to improve the quality of your complexion is by changing your eating habits. Surgery will create dramatic results (after a painful recovery) on the surface of the skin. However, the cause of aging and unsightly skin conditions goes much deeper and can be addressed with less aggressive means.

Supply oils and high-quality essential fatty acids from the inside out.

Hydrogenated and processed vegetable oils have replaced the intake of more fragile and nutritionally viable oils. Every cell of the body has a membrane that needs high-quality essential fatty acids to be maintained. Make sure your diet includes several of the following oil sources, cold-pressed and organic wherever possible: olive, sesame, sunflower, flax, borage, evening primrose, and fish oils.

Moderate, reduce, and eliminate the consumption of known toxins and stressors.

We have been conditioned to consider certain toxins as normal components of our modern diet. Caffeine, tobacco, alcohol, refined sugars and grains, pesticides, preservatives, and genetically modified foods are not normal nutritional compounds for us to process. They may be familiar and convenient, but they add stress to the body. This stress will ultimately be reflected on your face.

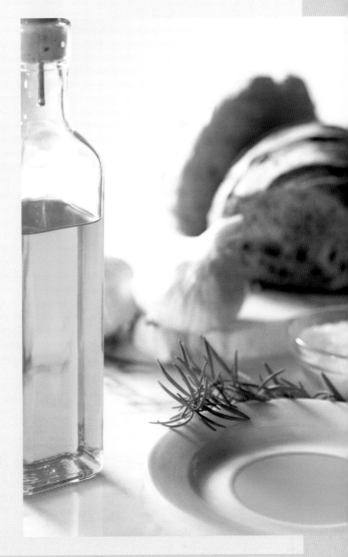

On any given day, we make hundreds of choices. But just how do we make these choices? From food and drink, to movies and books, from friends and family, to career and relationships, we are in a constant process, evaluating both our short- and long-term needs. In each moment, we can choose to nourish and replenish ourselves, or not. We decide what to eat and drink; how and when to move our bodies; when to rest, play, or work; when to sing, praise, blame, surrender, forgive; when to stop and take a deep breath; when to connect to the source that animates all of life and let life flow more deeply within us.

The good-better-best guideline will help you choose what is best in any given moment. The key factor in moving from good to better or better to best is a matter of life force. Choose to nourish yourself with that which has the most life force. The inherent life force in a substance or choice of activity will bring commensurate aliveness, vibrancy, and alignment to all levels of your being. It will nourish all of you, not just one part. Finishing the entire container of ice cream may feel good but saving some for tomorrow may be better. Reading until 2:00 A.M. may feel good, but getting the sleep you need for an early morning meeting may be better. Having another glass of wine during a stressful gathering may feel good, but leaving the gathering early instead is probably best.

We all know that drinking water is essential. When we choose a beverage, tap water is good if the alternative is drinking sweetened soda. Bottled water is better (given the amount of toxic chemicals in municipal water systems). The best choice is to have a water filtration system in your home and use it for all your drinking and cooking needs. Each of these simple choices—less sugar, more sleep, less wine, more water—has far-reaching implications for the efficacy of our metabolic functions, our blood sugar maintenance, and our emotional stability.

Consider the whole of your life, the situation, and the moment. Some days are best begun by nourishing your spirit with quiet time. Other days you best address your physical needs first with a morning stretch. Choose maximum life force in all you eat, drink, breathe, or do. That life force feeds the spark of the source that animates all life. It will give you more life with which to live. Once in balance, each part will add reflexively to the whole, and your life will become richer and more fulfilling.

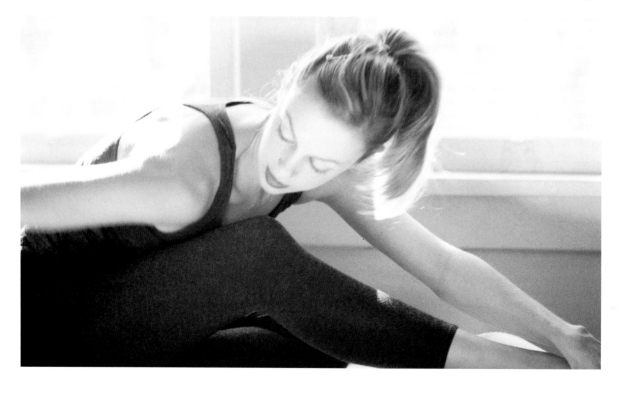

From the crown of the head to the soles of the feet, we exist within the miracle of the body. Its magnificence, complexity, efficiency, and grace elicit wonder and awe. In optimal health or physical crisis, contemplate the workings of your body for a moment and consider these mind-boggling numbers:

The body contains more than 100,000 miles (160,000 km) of blood vessels. The heart, approximately the size of your fist, beats 70 times per minute, more than 100,800 times a day, moving about 8 tons of blood in and out of its chambers. The total surface area of the alveoli (air sacs) in your lungs exceeds 20,000 square inches (130,000 sq cm). We inhale and exhale approximately 17 times per minute or 17,000 breaths per day. The nervous system, including minute neural branches, exceeds 10 million nerve fibers in constant communication. The skeleton contains 266 bones, all delicately adjusted to support the weight of skin and internal organs and the movement of more than 500 muscles. The 32-foot (10 m) long alimentary canal processes an average of 5.5 pounds (2.5 kg) of food and liquid each day. This amounts to 1 ton (0.9 metric ton) of solid and liquid nourishment annually.

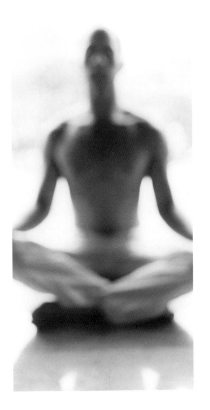

Our bodies perform these functions for us every second of every minute of every hour of every day of our lives. Amazingly, our bodies do this with virtually no conscious input from us. We depend on the body to take care of itself while we go on about our business. Often only at times of physical breakdown or faulty functioning do we appreciate the daily miracles that have been occurring all along. The body has the innate intelligence to build, repair, eliminate, and regenerate cells in its own perfect time and rhythm. The body does depend on us, however, to provide the raw materials to make this possible.

How to support the body in creating ultimate health and beauty is a complex and personal journey. As multidimensional beings, our health, our vitality, and our enthusiasm for life spring from a multifaceted interplay of factors—genetic, biological, karmic, and environmental. When we make choices, we do not just consider our bodies. We also weigh the needs of our emotions, our minds, our pocketbooks, our comforts, and our convenience. Some choices are positive and support us on all levels: a soothing cup of tea, a long walk, a quiet time of prayer or meditation, a much-needed conversation with a friend. Some are relatively negative and can be detrimental to one or more levels of our being: the third latte of the day, a couch potato weekend, bar hopping with our friends. We make different choices in different situations, and we reap the benefits or suffer the consequences accordingly. With just a few simple changes or additions, we can bring greater vitality to our body and immediately infuse life-enhancing vibrancy to all aspects of our life.

Consider these basic guidelines to help you make choices on a physical level that will affect all other levels of being. Evaluate the quality of your four priority sources of energy, consider the principles of rejuvenating nutrition, review your daily needs and choose the best you can for yourself.

DETOXIFICATION AND ELIMINATION

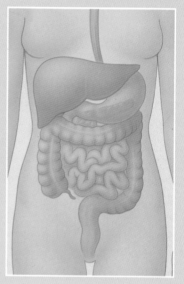

Nothing happens in the body without the organs and systems working in close cooperation with one another. Usually, we think of breathing taking place in the lungs and eating taking place in the mouth. However, respiration and assimilation of nutrients also take place on the cellular level. The respiratory system filters the air, but the circulatory system carries oxygen and carbon dioxide to and from the cells. We process food and water through the digestive system, but the liver and the kidneys purify the nutrients and prepare them to be transported again by the blood to the cells. Elimination of unused raw material and metabolic wastes are excreted via the kidneys (liquid) or the colon (solids). Finally, the largest organ of purification and elimination, the skin, supports each of these organs and functions in surprisingly effective ways.

Supporting the organs of detoxification and elimination, using the good-better-best guideline, and following the principles of rejuvenating nutrition will enhance the body's overall performance. Radiant health is the reflection of care and awareness of our complete selves.

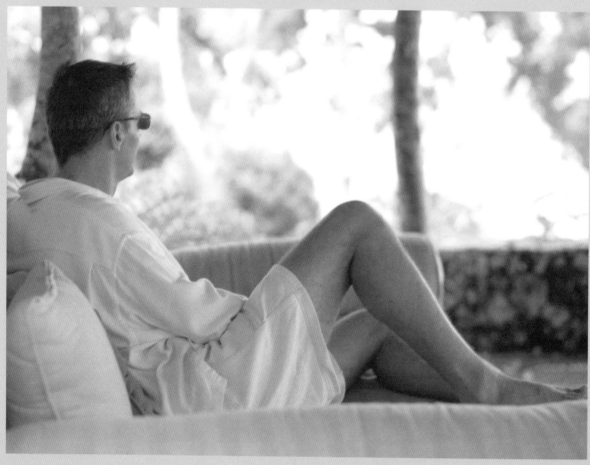

Lungs

All living beings depend upon cyclic breathing to maintain their existence. Animals (including humans) and plants use the waste products of each other's respiratory cycles to live. The Sun takes what scientists call a breath (solar wind) every 11 years. On average, we inhale 35 pounds (16 kg) of oxygen on a daily basis (six times the amount of food and water combined) and exhale carbon dioxide and small amounts of water.

Oxygen is needed to convert nutrients chemically into energy and to eliminate toxins on the cellular level. Lack of oxygen causes poor metabolism of food and allows bacteria to proliferate in the blood. Oxygen maintains metabolic functions bodywide, calming the nervous system, allowing the brain to process billions of bits of data, purifying the blood, and enhancing immune functions. Deep breathing is given a higher priority as a source of energy than is food because the increase in oxygen through breathing releases energy for immediate use.

Kidneys

Our kidneys, suspended near our spine and just below the ribs and weighing merely 1 pound (0.5 kg) total, filter our entire blood supply more than 400 times each day. Every time the heart beats, 20 percent of the blood is filtered through this system. The kidneys regulate the inner sea and its concentration of minerals. Homeostasis on a cellular level is based on a delicate balance of chemicals suspended in a watery solution. To make a simple comparison, the body is like a bathtub of water with a handful of dissolved minerals wrapped in a nearly waterproof container. Mineral-rich water fills and surrounds our cells—70 percent of our body mass is water. Two-thirds of this water is found within the cells, and one-third makes up the fluid of our blood.

With infinite precision, the million tiny filters in each kidney maintain the homeostasis of the elements in the inner sea. The proportions are microscopic. However, when any ingredient increases or decreases, the kidneys are activated to rebalance the watery solution. They filter out what we do not need and prepare the waste for excretion as urine. The kidneys also recycle water, mineral salts, and sugars back into the bloodstream to meet the body's moment-to-moment needs. Lack of sufficient water results in sluggish blood, slowed filtration, and impaired kidney function. A simple solution to many aches and pains of body and mind is to drink more water.

Liver

The liver, located below the diaphragm on the right side of the body, is responsible for the purification of the bloodstream. It is the body's primary organ of detoxification. The liver prepares the blood to carry a maximum of nutrition and a minimum of toxins to every cell in the body. Before the heart pumps the blood to the body, the blood must be cleansed and purified to the best of the liver's ability.

The liver has more than 500 known functions. Making and secreting enzymes (over 3,000 catalyze over 7,000 chemical and metabolic processes in the body) is just one function. These enzymes are essential to neutralizing most drugs and environmental poisons that enter the body through food, drink, and air. They also carry out the basic metabolic functions that sustain life. The liver metabolizes essential fats and oils (cholesterol, triglycerides, lipoproteins and so on), thus preventing their accumulation on blood vessel walls (atherosclerosis). The liver also synthesizes necessary blood proteins and secretes bile to aid digestion.

The holistic prescription against processed foods, excessive chemicals (alcohol, nicotine, and caffeine), pesticides, and preservatives is based on the harmful assault of these chemicals on the hardworking liver. If the liver has the best possible raw material to work with, its detoxification load is reduced and its ability to support regeneration is greatly enhanced.

Colon

Elimination is as essential as ingestion. What we put into our bodies by way of food and drink is often a major preoccupation, perhaps even a primary avocation and delight. Yet little thought is given to the eliminative process until such time as it ceases to occur naturally. The 6-foot-long (2 m) colon, curled in a horseshoe shape around the small intestine, holds, prepares, and releases the solid matter that the body does not need. Without the easy, daily removal of unwanted, unneeded matter, the body would quickly pollute itself, filling the bloodstream with toxins and offering poor nutrition to the cells. The liver, kidneys, lungs, and skin would be significantly stressed.

Dietary choices impact the colon and thus the quality of the blood and every cell. The colon requires a diet rich in natural-fiber foods (whole grains and vegetables), fruits to cleanse, healthy oils to lubricate, and plenty of water to move things along.

The skin is a vast, complex, semi-permeable membrane measuring about 18 square feet (1.6 sq m), that defines the body in physical space. It is the barrier of protection between the elements of nature and the life-sustaining processes within the body. It is the body's first line of defense from injury. To work well, the skin must remain elastic and supple, the pores responsive to the needs of the moment, the nerves alert and catalyzed.

The tendency to disassociate the human exterior from matters of bodily health is most curious considering the scope of the skin's functions. Our chief concern seems to be to adorn it, using it as a showcase for the personality. Our appearance is important to our emotional and mental health. However, the skin is actually an impressive mirror of the internal terrain and the status of biochemical functioning. As the body's largest organ of elimination, it bears the detoxification load whenever the liver, kidney, colon, and lung functions are compromised. Skin disorders—acne, eruptions, boils, unusual odors, excessive sweating, psoriasis, or eczema—signal the overload of toxic conditions elsewhere in the body. We treat the skin as single layer. Instead it is an intricate tri-level structure with multiple functions performed by the epidermis, the dermis, and the subcutaneous fatty layer. In 1 square inch (6.5 sq cm) of skin are found fully 3 feet (1 m) of blood vessels, 20 hairs, 12 feet (4 m) of nerve fibers with 25 nerve endings, 100 sweat glands, and 30 oil glands—in total more than 3 million cells. Yet at no point is the skin more than $3/16$ of an inch (0.5 cm) thick.

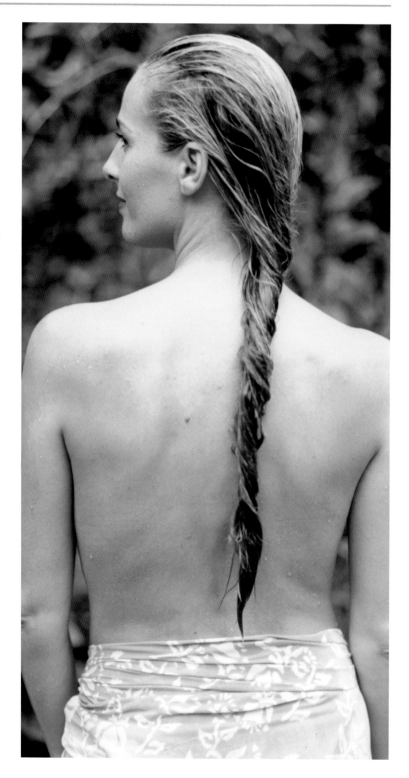

Epidermis

The outer layer of the skin is the epidermis, a flattened protein substance called keratin. The epidermis provides the durable, waterproof shell of protection that surrounds our body. The epidermal skin cells have a self-renewing life cycle. Old cells are sloughed off naturally as you soak in a bath, dry your body with a towel, rub your face, or sit in a chair. Exfoliation is necessary on a daily basis. This explains why 30 percent of the dust in our homes is made up of dead skin cells.

The epidermis is approximately 12–15 cell layers deep. New round skin cells are born in the deeper layers, close to the dermis, and push upward to the outer layer. As they rise, they begin to flatten and dry out, helping to contain the moisture in the lower layers of the skin and the body. When they reach the surface, they spread out to form a scaly, shingled layer of protection. This older, hardened (keratinized) outer layer is constantly sloughed off and renewed. The regenerative ability of the skin is called upon whenever the skin is pierced, cut, or bruised. New cells immediately proliferate as the skin mends itself. The remarkable healing ability of our skin is our primary insurance against severe injury, germs, and infection.

This top layer of the epidermis is comprised of dead skin cells. Rather than useless cells to be removed as quickly as possible, these dead cells are adapted to protect the body in different ways. For one, the body transforms them into a transparent windshield over the cornea, allowing light to enter the retina and further shielding the cornea with the delicate outer eyelid. Epidermal cells also form thicker deposits as nails on the tips of the nerve-sensitive fingers and toes, create tiny ridges on the fingertips to provide traction, and build up calluses to counter the wear and tear of pressure points on the hands and feet. The epidermis also softens into pleats to allow joint flexibility.

When we are in our 20s, 30s, and 40s, this process of renewal takes approximately three weeks. By the time we reach our mid-50s, the process has slowed down to six to eight weeks. The current cosmetic rage of glycolic and alpha hydroxy acid peels forces faster and unnaturally deep exfoliation as a solution to aging, wrinkled skin. What seems like a solution, however, can impede the skin's natural ability to renew itself. Most topical, aggressive, and speedy solutions are only temporary and can damage the tender layers of skin, permanently affecting their functions.

Dermis

This deeper middle layer of skin teems with activity. It contains all the structures that we associate with the skin: nerve endings, tiny blood and lymph vessels, hair follicles, pores, sweat glands, and oil glands. The dermis receives and transmits sensory stimuli to the brain as nerve impulses, regulates body temperature through perspiration, and produces protein fibers (collagen and elastin) to maintain the skin's protective resilience and youthful bounce.

The structure of the skin functions through absorption and secretion. In a limited fashion, the skin absorbs whatever substances are applied to it, whether nutritive or toxic. Your choice of skin care and bathing products is important to your body's health. A good guideline is that if you would not want to eat or drink a product, you do not want to put it onto your skin or into your bath.

The skin also releases metabolic toxins, oils, and water. By releasing toxic-bearing fluids and metabolic wastes through perspiration, the skin assists the other organs of elimination in detoxifying the body. The secretions from your sweat and oil glands provide your skin's acid mantle—a thin film of perspiration and oil that lubricates and softens the skin as it provides a primary barrier to bacterial and viral infections. Many commercial products harshly strip the skin of these natural oils, thus damaging the necessary acid mantle.

Subcutaneous Fatty Layer

Below the epidermis and dermis is a layer of fatty tissue. These fat cells are essential to our beauty and our health. The fatty layer protects the internal organs, stores nutrients, retains internal heat, and provides added resiliency to the other layers of the skin.

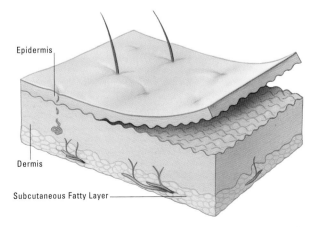

Epidermis

Dermis

Subcutaneous Fatty Layer

DETOX AND PURIFICATION

The ultimate key to cellular and systemic detoxification is proper nourishment for the body. If you give your body the best air, water, and food that you can, it will receive and absorb the new nutrients and naturally let go of stored toxins and metabolic wastes. Unfortunately, the body, mind, and heart deal with far more stress than the physical mechanism is capable of handling without showing some distress. When we lighten the load on the body's systems of purification and detoxification, we strengthen our life energy.

External beauty is the result of an inner process. Inner beauty is a functional experience. The cells are free of toxins, the emotions are balanced, the mind is calm, the spirit is at peace. With all levels in harmony, we have the energy we need to meet the often overwhelming demands of the external world. Responding with grace and ease arises from this level of purification. This is inner transformation with external beauty as the result—a natural face-lift.

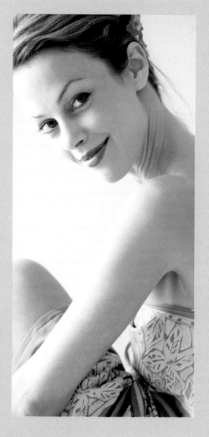

The suggestions throughout this text are designed to aid cellular detoxification in a gentle manner. They are not quick fixes or magic pills. Consistency and dedication are needed to help the cells of the body function at an optimal level. Make changes slowly and at your own pace. In an ideal world, we would have time to focus on each of the four priority sources of energy daily. We would spend time increasing our connection with spirit, use our favorite breathing practices to oxygenate the body several times a day, drink more than eight glasses of pure water effortlessly, and eat food that is vibrant and alive throughout the day. Pick and choose to incorporate the suggestions and the rituals from the other chapters to increase your vitality while focusing on self-nurturing on all levels.

DRY SKIN BRUSHING

One of the simplest ways to exfoliate the dead skin cells from the whole body is dry skin brushing. This process can begin or end the day, detoxify cold or flu symptoms, or energize the whole system in fewer than ten minutes. Dry skin brushing stimulates lymph and blood circulation, activates the oil glands, tones the skin, and supports the adrenal glands.

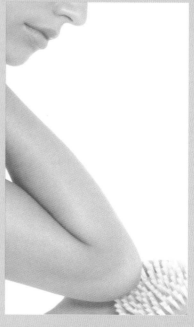

Procedure

1. Use a vegetable bristle brush (available in most health food stores).
2. Apply the brush to bare, dry skin in patterns that follow the flow of lymph and blood.
3. Brush from the extremities toward the heart, from the upper torso down, and from the lower abdomen up.
4. Use long, gentle brush strokes or small circular motions as inspired.
5. Listen to your body; some areas will request gentle sweeps while other parts demand more vigorous sweeps.

HONI-VIN

For generations, the combination of honey and vinegar has been a superb addition to a healthy diet. A glass sipped at mealtime greatly aids digestion and restores the body's natural acid-alkaline balance. A glass taken during times of stress will renew your harmony in the moment and give you the emotional stability to deal with life's challenges. Honi-Vin is a high-vitamin and mineral cocktail filled with enzymes to balance you physically and emotionally.

1. Blend equal amounts of unheated, organic honey with organic apple cider vinegar. This will be your concentrate. Create a mix that tastes good to you by adding a little more honey or vinegar.
2. Keep the concentrate in a well-sealed bottle or jar. It can be stored for months and still retain its potency.
3. To make a Honi-Vin drink, add concentrate to water (hot or cold). Start with 1 teaspoon in a cup and build up to several tablespoons.
4. Make it as strong or as weak as you like, allowing your taste buds to determine what is right for you at any given moment.
OPTIONAL: Add some powdered cayenne pepper to stimulate circulation and sharpen your mind.

INNER GUIDANCE

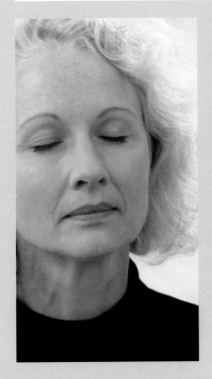

The guidelines in this book are simply guidelines. You are your own best resource. Detoxification can happen on any level of being: cleaning out the closet; being willing to let go of old thoughts, feelings, and behaviors; recreating a spiritual practice; or simply bringing the body's chemistry back into balance are all elements of detox.

1. Sit quietly and do the heart breath (Chapter 6).
2. Add the Rejuv Breath (Chapter 4), and connect to your heart.
3. Ask for the help you need to detox and recover your full vibrancy and well-being.
4. Repeat the heart breath as you listen for inspiration.
5. Act on what you hear, see, or feel is right for you.
6. Repeat this process often as a way to build your personal relationship with the spirit within.

BODY BREW TEA

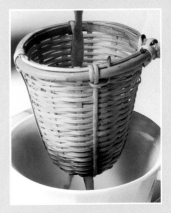

Make a pot and drink it throughout the day to renew and detoxify all major systems of the body.
1. Make a stock bottle of this dried herb combination: equal parts by volume of organic yarrow blossoms, red raspberry leaves, mullein leaves, and nettles.
2. Store in a glass container away from direct sunlight. To make two cups of tea, use 2 heaped teaspoons of the blend.
3. Pour 2 cups (500 ml) of boiling water over the herbs and steep, covered, for ten minutes.
4. Strain (not through aluminum), and sweeten to taste.
5. Drink warm or cool throughout the day.

3. POINTS OF CONSCIOUSNESS

LIFE AT ITS FULLEST IS A FLEXIBLE DANCE BETWEEN POLARITIES—DIVINE AND HUMAN, FEMALE AND MALE, LEFT AND RIGHT, OPEN AND CLOSED, STILLNESS AND MOTION. ARE WE SPIRITUAL BEINGS HAVING A PHYSICAL EXPERIENCE OR PHYSICAL BEINGS HAVING A SPIRITUAL EXPERIENCE? WHERE ARE YOU ON THIS CONTINUUM? WE WILL EXPLORE OUR UNIQUE SELVES WITHIN THE COSMIC DANCE OF PARTICLES AND ENERGIES.

In Rejuv, we regard the head with wonder and reverence as the access point to the fullness of being. The cranium protects a complex and sophisticated machine—the brain—the physical point of registry for all senses, feelings, and thoughts. Rejuv uses the ancient healing art of reflexology to touch specific areas on the face and head, also known as nerve center points. Each of these centers is a living system, unique to each individual, in flux from moment to moment. The Rejuv Touch activates the innate intelligence of each center and synchronizes communication throughout the body using the principles of reflexology. This activation helps to realign the body's physical and energetic systems.

The Rejuv pathways are multidimensional channels between the central core of energy in the body and the flow of energy that moves out to our periphery. By sweeping the pathways, we are able to clear the emotional crystallizations that have built up over time and to rejuvenate the flow of life force in these channels. The energy can be locked into any level of our being. However, once released, it can flow into a refreshed pathway to a nerve center where it will either be reintegrated or be dissipated completely. This renewed energy flow not only enlivens the bones, muscles, blood, lymph, and nerves of the face but also supports the vibrancy of the chakra system.

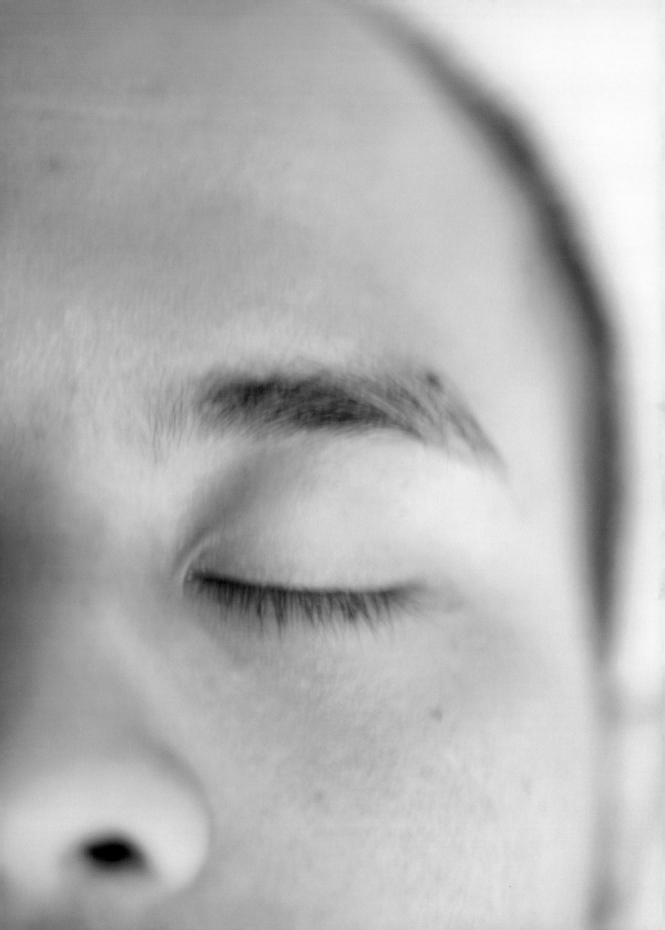

LIFE'S ESSENTIALS

Human curiosity compels us to explore the nature of our world and ourselves. We want to know who and what we are. We live in a world of substances—solids, liquids, and gases—all made of tiny particles, called atoms. Atoms, or elements, bond together to form molecules. Molecules join other molecules in specific groups and chains to form compounds. These basic elements combine to create everything we recognize—water, wood, steel, food, even our own bodies.

Science has penetrated the atom and its structures. Each element is actually made up of even smaller bits of matter—the nucleus (protons and neutrons) with electrons spinning in orbital rings. Quantum physics has looked even deeper and found even smaller bits, such as quarks, mesons, and neutrinos. Instead of finding the smallest particle of matter, a new reality has emerged. What has always seemed solid is actually vast empty space and what seemed to be tiny particles are actually aggregates of energy with probability of motion.

Imagine enlarging the nucleus of an atom from your body to the size of a head on a straight pin. Just to see it, we would need to magnify it many billions of times. You would find the first ring of electrons approximately 30 feet (10 m) away from you. The nucleus can be likened to a speck floating in an empty room, with the electrons spinning outside the room. How do we live in a world of substance when all the solid building blocks are filled with energy and empty space?

Each human being is a unique signature of molecules. When we refer to the substance of our being, our other bodies are not just concepts, they are real and substantial. Our physical body is the densest aggregate of our atomic reality. We live in our physical bodies but also have varied states of being that spin or vibrate at different frequencies.

Our energy body, a lighter version of our physical body, vibrates at a higher frequency and spins a little faster than the dense physical body. This energy body is palpable. It moves in and through our physical body but takes up a little more space—about 2 inches (5 cm) beyond the skin. Our health depends on the ability of these two bodies (energetic and physical) to maintain their equilibrium and nourish one other.

We have many ways to support our physical structures. An alternative healing modality may be needed to support the well-being of the energetic body.

Humans are feeling beings. Feelings are among the purest spiritual experiences we can have. The feeling body vibrates a little faster and extends a little farther from the energetic and physical bodies. The feeling body is the direct connection to intuition, inner knowing, and gut feelings. We often rush to interpret, label, and categorize these feeling tones into emotional story lines, thus losing their essential messages. As we learn to listen to the feeling tones, we can access inner guidance and bypass information from our personal biases and past experiences.

Extending beyond the feeling body, not limited by the physical brain, is the mind. The concrete sequential mind can follow a plan. It gives us the ability to bake a cake or fly to the Moon. The concrete mind is complemented by the creative mind, the source of the brilliant fire of ideas rising from nothing. These two aspects of mind penetrate all the other levels, spin a little faster, take up more space. We can be so lost in thought that we miss the exit on the freeway. This is not the best way to drive a car, perhaps, but an example of the depth and breath of our multidimensional abilities.

Our spiritual body—the fastest spinning body—penetrates all the other bodies and stands out farther still, seemingly invisible to our senses. This body is the animating principle of our being. It is the aspect of each of us that has always been and always will be. Depending on your preference of terms, this is the body of your highest self, divine self, or soul.

We are the dance of spirit coalescing into thought, feeling, energy, and atoms. Our thoughts affect our feelings, our energy, and our physicality. When the physical body hurts, our energy, feelings, and thoughts are affected. There is no separation. We are multilayered bodies creating a wholeness of being. The essence permeating every single molecule is our unique signature.

In the reality of this vast empty space, transformation—physiological, energetic, emotional, mental, and spiritual—is possible. The Rejuv Touch is applied to the face and head to access this space for transformation on every level of being.

Reflexology is an ancient science and a healing art based on the principle that certain areas of the body (feet, hands, and head) contain reflex points that correspond to the body's organs, systems, and tissues:

• The most well-known system is foot reflexology, an incredibly effective tool for both chronic and acute conditions and first aid in the right hands at the right time.

• Hands are more accessible but the reflexology points are less familiar and rarely used.

• Head reflexology is rarer still, but it is perhaps the most powerful reflex map of all.

These reflex systems function in unique ways. Our feet move, support, and connect us to the Earth. They provide balance, equilibrium, and mobility like no other part of our body. Our hands let us touch the world around us. We use them to reach out, touch, create, shape, receive, and communicate. The mind initiates, directs, and registers all our interactions, within and without, through our brain and sensory organs. When we work with the whole-body maps of reflexology, we create both physical and metaphorical changes. Not only is our physiology touched and shifted, but we also enliven the qualities that the areas represent energetically, emotionally, mentally, and spiritually.

HeadWise reflexology can help us to access our executive ability, or what our brain is telling our body to do even before we do it. The brain is the point of registry for all of the sensory input we receive from our five senses and process through the neurological networks of the brain. Our experiences are filtered, arranged, and registered to create our unique perception of the world. When the physical and spiritual systems are in sync, we often have greater access to clear vision, clear hearing,

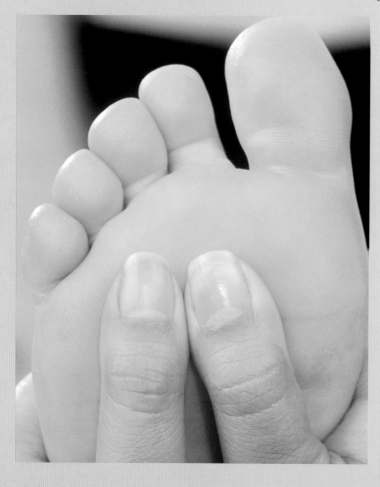

clear knowing, and clear action. These skills are not psychic gifts but natural capacities that are hardwired into the body.

The Rejuv Touch philosophy regards the head with reverence because it is the key to accessing a person's core identity. The head houses and protects the delicate mass of neurological matter—the brain—the primary point of registry within us for all we have experienced. This is the place that stores all we are, all we have been, and all we have longed to be. It is just beneath our fingertips as we provide loving intentionality through the Rejuv Touch.

As we touch the head, we are fully aware that its reflex points affect every single system of the body. We use the Rejuv rituals, nerve center points, and pathways to nourish all the levels of being. Touching the head in this sacred way acknowledges the spirit, stills the mind, and calms the emotions. The flow of energies through the head is refreshed, the metabolic functions throughout the brain and body are enhanced, and our faces reveal the ease and radiance of a natural face-lift.

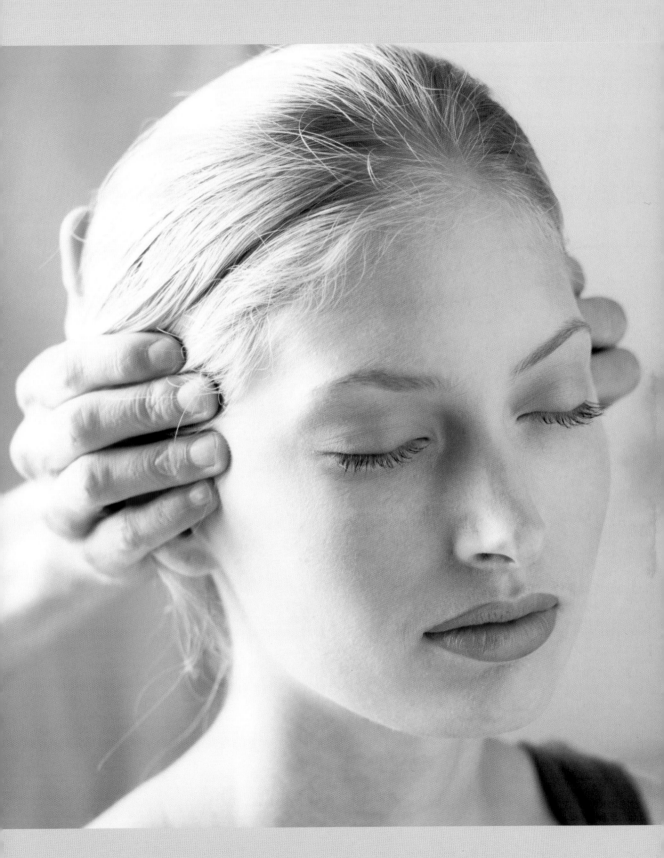

As we approach the nerve centers and pathways employed in the Rejuv Touch, some common reference points will facilitate accurate location of these areas. The coronal plane divides the body into posterior and anterior (back and front), while the midsagittal plane (midline) divides the body laterally (left and right), thus creating four quadrants. These planes are shown on the images below as lines. The nerve center points are located in reference to the planes. The pathways follow the contour of the bones from the midline to the coronal plane.

In Rejuv, we consider these planes not as mere anatomical convention but as physical condensation of light and life force— a vibrant substance that supports alignment and communication between all five levels of being. These two planes intersect at the spinal column and chakra system to create a central core of light structure. The Rejuv pathways flow from the midline to the coronal plane, from the core to the periphery.

Based on the principles of reflexology, the work we do in one area affects the entire system. Rejuv movements begin at the midline of the face and sweep to the sides. When we work the front quadrants of the face in this way, we open and expand reflexively the front quadrants of the body and the back quadrants of the head and body. As we open and uplift the physical structures, we open the ornament of our light structures, refreshing the flow of the life force providing more vitality and radiance to all levels of being.

Picture an inexpensive decorative ornament—a wedding bell, a pumpkin, an Easter egg—created out of colored tissue and two pieces of cardboard that unfold to reveal the honeycomb of paper that creates a three-dimensional form. To a child's eye, it seems like magic. Whenever we do a sweep from midline to coronal, we magically and reflexively open the light ornament—the core of our being—360 degrees.

MIDSAGITTAL (MIDLINE) PLANE

CORONAL PLANE

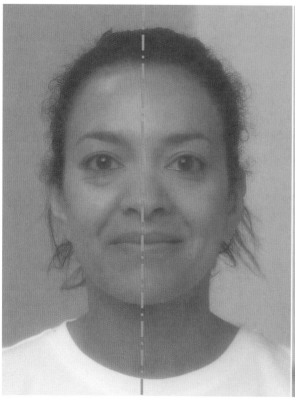
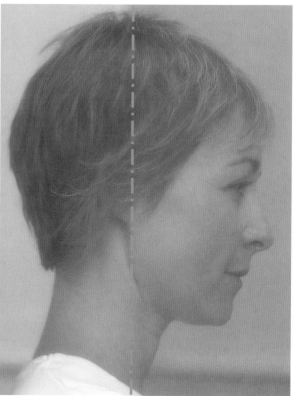

THE TREAD AND RISER

To facilitate the placement of your fingertips and pads, imagine a stairwell. If the step is the tread, what holds up each step is the riser. The bony structures of the face may also be designated as treads and risers. The treads of the cheeks and forehead are the broad expanses of each area. Where the tread becomes the riser is an edge. In many rituals, this edge marks the location for the sweep.

The cleft and the hollow are two other prominent locations.

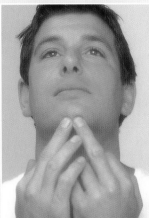

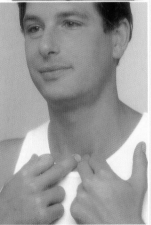

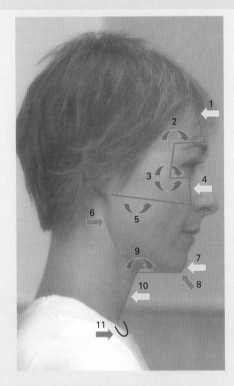

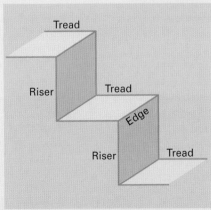

KEY

1. Tread of the forehead

2. Upper riser of the orbital ridge

3. Riser lower orbital ridge and upper cheekbone

4. Tread of the cheekbone

5. Lower riser of the cheekbone

6. Ramus of the jaw

7. Tread of the jaw

8. Cleft of the chin

9. Riser of the jaw and neck

10. Tread of the neck

11. The neck hollow

CHIN—CLEFT

The midline of the chin is called the cleft. Rejuv work on the jawbone encompasses the tread, the riser, the edge, and the cleft.

NECK—HOLLOW

Neck work always begins at the hollow (the sternal notch) sweeping up the tread of the neck, along the riser of the jaw, around the ramus, to the parotid point.

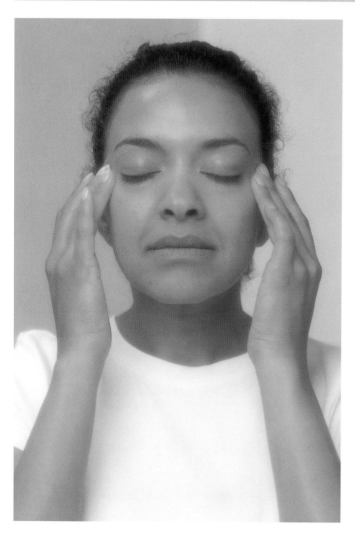

A gentle touch at the temple points empowers the innate intelligence of the nerve centers.

The Rejuv nerve centers are living systems, islands of consciousness unique to each individual. They adjust to each moment and respond to the essence of life force moving through them. Within the vastness of subatomic space, these centers of cohesion are where all the levels of being meet and clear communication between them is enhanced.

Imagine that these major nerve centers are like the Grand Central Station or Waterloo of a whole being. At these stations, trains come in, passengers get off, passengers get on, and trains move out to their destinations. This network of rails, scheduling, and staffing transports thousands of people in relative comfort and safety every day over hundreds of miles. This is a complex system, to be sure. Nothing, though, compares with the body's system where the living energies from all of our bodies come together, communicate and relay information, and then move outward again. Nerve centers are where the incoming energies are sorted, cataloged, and redirected. The energies move out to their designated destinations and purposes for perfect use and balance.

Each nerve center is innately intelligent and has the capacity to assess the energy flowing through itself. It knows whether an energetic substance is nourishing and appropriate for the individual body and being. It also recognizes when a substance is not nourishing or when a particular holding pattern is no longer appropriate. Each nerve center evaluates energetic substances (emotions, thought patterns, psychological behaviors, muscular contractions or extensions, and so on) and determines whether or not they are appropriate at any given moment. Nerve centers consider our needs on many levels instantly, integrating, assimilating, or dissipating the energy.

A gentle touch at a nerve center empowers the center's innate intelligence to activate, synchronize, and refresh the flow between our physical, energetic, emotional, mental, and spiritual bodies. These points respond quickly to the influx of life force from our hands and hearts. As we touch these living islands of consciousness, they shift and change in tone, feeling, and even location, however minutely, adjusting themselves constantly into balance and wholeness. Working with the Rejuv Touch (see Chapter 4) on these nerve centers is a communicative, connective, and cocreative process.

LOCATION AND FUNCTION OF NERVE CENTERS

The nerve centers are physical areas where blood, nerve, and lymph channels may be found in close proximity. They are not simply nerve access points. Use the following illustrations and descriptions as a general map to locate them on your face. However, rely on your fingertips to fine-tune your position by sensing a buzzing, a warm tingling feeling that indicates just the right place. Follow your intuition and subtle perceptions. Over time, these living systems will respond to your touch and your fingertips will seem to sink into the points with ease.

Specific directions are provided with each ritual. As a general rule, there is no heavy pressure. Your touch should be featherlight, tender, and receptive. Each time you reach a nerve center, hold the point in a moment of stillness. Each hold is a moment of activation, synchronization, or integration. Take time to hold a space for yourself, acknowledge your conscious intention, and pause to be with your whole being.

Adjusting our internal flows is a multi-leveled task because we are the composite of multiple frequencies of energies. Within the vast spacious emptiness of our sub-atomic being, it truly is possible to smooth a jagged shape or to alter a rough texture. At its core, the Rejuv Touch is about this level of transformation.

Location of the nerve centers with the lines of intersection for the location of the temple points.

KEY

- Crown
- Pituitary
- Temple
- Nose
- Mouth corner
- Parotid
- Triangle ear
— Temple intersection

SIDE VIEW OF NERVE CENTERS   FRONT VIEW OF NERVE CENTERS

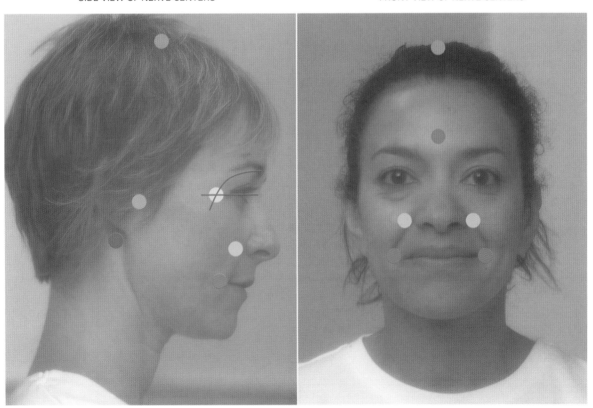

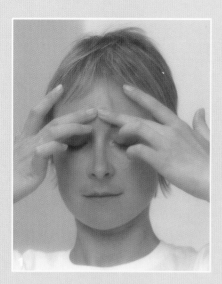

2. NOSE POINTS

LOCATION: The nose points are located at the side of the widest point of the flair of each nostril. The fingertips should point directly (not angled) into the cheekbone when you hold these points.

FUNCTION: Held in stillness, these points relax the diaphragm, in turn relaxing both the lungs and the heart. As the diaphragmatic muscle relaxes, it triggers a release of tension in all the organs that touch it, both above and below: heart, lungs, liver, stomach, pancreas, and spleen. The nose points energize the muscles of the cheeks, preparing the pathway for an abundant free flow of energy.

3. MOUTH CORNER POINTS

LOCATION: Mouth corner points are found just at the corners of the lips. Fingertips should touch both the corner of the lips and the muscle just beyond on either side.

FUNCTION: These points help release holding patterns in the soft tissue systems of the pelvis and lower abdomen: bladder, uterus, rectum, and sex organs. Energetically, they reflex the first and second chakras softening tissues of survival, sexuality, and creativity. They allow locked energies in the muscles and tissues of the lips and surrounding area to release all the things you did not have the courage to say and wish you had, as well as all the things you did say and wish you had not.

1. PITUITARY POINT

LOCATION: The pituitary point is located on the midline of the forehead, just above the space between the brows. Place both index fingertips (or middle fingertips) side by side on the point.

FUNCTION: Holding the pituitary point prepares the body to accept change and to utilize and ground healing energy on a cellular level. This point stimulates the pituitary gland, the physical plant manager of the body. It tells the body what to do, when to do it, and how to do it. This master gland manages all the hormonal signals of the body. The pituitary and pineal glands work together to assist in the healthy functioning of the third eye.

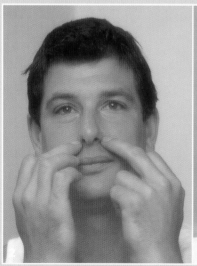
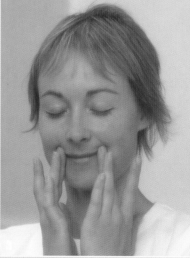
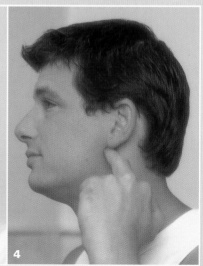

4. PAROTID POINTS

LOCATION: The parotid point is a soft hollow that usually falls just below the earlobe at the juncture between the jawbone (mandible) and the ear bone (mastoid). Place fingertips into the hollows.

FUNCTION: The parotids are salivary glands located in the cheeks. These points assist energetic and physical digestion. The gland itself works with the essence of food—what nourishes and what depletes the body—as well as how we digest our food and our life experiences. Physically, it assists the brain in preparing appropriate digestive enzymes. Spiritually, it aids us in the assimilation of minerals and light.

5. TRIANGLE EAR POINTS

LOCATION: The triangle ear points are the little hollows just in front of each ear. Find the triangle-shaped cartilage protecting the ear canal and place your fingertip in the hollow between the cartilage and the jawbone.

FUNCTION: The triangle-shaped cartilage protects the opening of the ear. This nerve center will reorder and balance the musculature and connective tissue of the jaw and cheekbone area, help relieve temporomandibular joint (TMJ) tension, and ease ear disharmonies. It will also refine your auditory perceptions: physically, your ability to hear sound; spiritually, your capacity to listen to others and to the world around you.

6. TEMPLE POINTS

LOCATION: The precise location of each temple point is at the intersection of two extended lines—a horizontal line from the pupil beyond the outer corner of the eye and the curved line down from the end of the eye brows. Place fingertips into the shallow indentation of the bone slightly beyond the orbital ridge.

FUNCTION: These points release the sutures between the bones that comprise this area—the frontal, temporal, and sphenoid bones. As the tension is released from each of these sutures, all of the cranial sutures also release, allowing fresh blood and lymph flow to the brain and spinal cord. The eyes and all their structures are refreshed. The pituitary is also activated when these points are stimulated.

7. CROWN POINT

LOCATION: The crown point is located at the top of the head in the center of the crown chakra (where the soft spot was during infancy). To locate this point, place the heel of one hand onto the bridge of the nose and align the middle finger on the midline; this fingertip will be touching the crown point.

FUNCTION: This point stimulates the pineal gland, the plant manager of the spiritual and energetic body. Physically, the pineal gland produces melatonin, which regulates the sleep cycle. Energetically, it assimilates spiritual and cosmic energies, strengthening the interface between all levels of being.

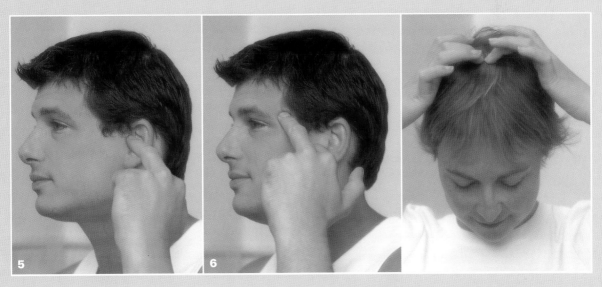

If the nerve centers are the train stations of the bodily system, the Rejuv pathways are the rails. In order for life energies to move smoothly within and between all bodies, the pathways must be clear and flowing. When the flow is unimpeded, the physical and energetic systems are aligned and we function with greater ease and a sense of wholeness.

Primarily, the Rejuv pathways flow between two planes of energy—the uplifting, vertical, midsagittal plane and the expanding, lateral, coronal plane. Obviously, our bodies are comprised of more than these two planes. Energy flows spirally, diagonally, horizontally, and in all directions in between. These energy flows are a complex matrix of meridians, as sophisticated as any of our biological systems—blood, lymph, and nerve.

Since we are multidimensional beings, an impact in any one area affects the entire system. When a contraction occurs within a pathway, the flow of life force is impeded. Usually, these tiny emotional crystallizations are created, released, and reintegrated into the system without our conscious participation. However, over time, recurring judgments, habitual responses, and holding patterns can overburden the pathways, clog the natural flow, and affect the tone of our musculature and the functioning of our internal organs. The quality of touch we use on our bodies and our faces will dictate the response of all the variegated tissues, affect how they function, regenerate, let go of toxins and uptake nutrition both physically and energetically.

Rejuv techniques encourage the outgoing flow through the pathways in their natural rhythm and direction from the core to the periphery. The movements of hands and fingers on the face initiate and support lateral (coronal) and vertical (midsagittal) expansions. The physical technique for this natural face-lift focuses on opening from midline to coronal.

The Rejuv process opens and clears, expands and refreshes the inherent pathways within the face and head. Continuous smoothing sweeps along the length of the pathways disturb and loosen emotional crystallizations. The released energy is then transported to a nerve center. Once these physical and energetic pathways are opened and reconnected to appropriate nerve centers, they offer a free flow of life force to the entire body, not just the face. Deep rest, renewal, and rejuvenation is experienced body-wide.

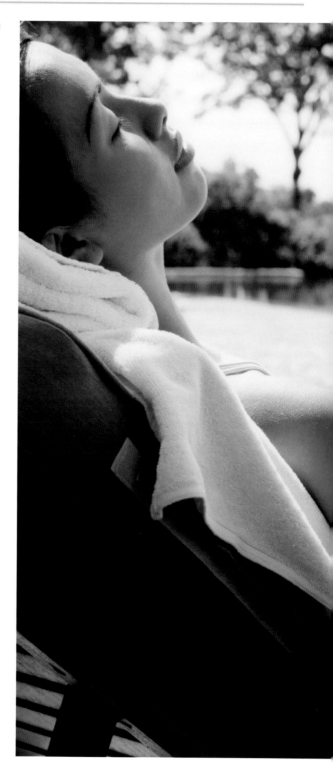

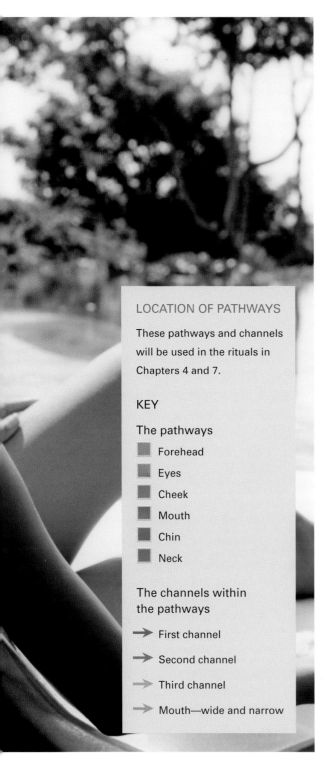

The function of the pathways is to transport clogged or stagnant energies to nerve centers to be processed properly. Cellular communication encourages cells to release holding patterns on any level. However, we need not be aware of the exact cause or location of the emotional crystallizations, whether a tight muscle, a stubborn thought, or an old emotion. We need only bring our care and attention to the pathways to enhance elasticity and regain connectivity within them. On the forehead, cheeks, mouth, and neck, the pathways have several distinct channels to access energy flow more precisely. Each pathway corresponds to a physical and metaphorical area of the face. The significance of each area will be described as we begin to use them in the Daily Rejuv Touch Ritual (Chapter 4) and in the advanced Rejuv techniques (Chapter 7).

LOCATION OF PATHWAYS

These pathways and channels will be used in the rituals in Chapters 4 and 7.

KEY

The pathways

■ Forehead

■ Eyes

■ Cheek

■ Mouth

■ Chin

■ Neck

The channels within the pathways

➜ First channel

➜ Second channel

➜ Third channel

➜ Mouth—wide and narrow

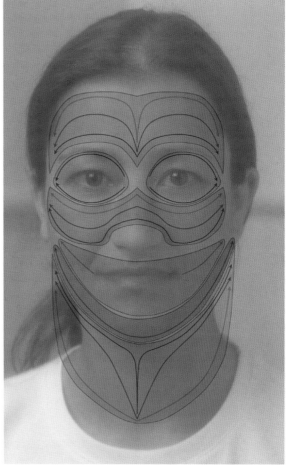

4. THE REJUV TOUCH

THE REJUV TOUCH IS A SIMPLE ART TECHNIQUE ELEVATED TO AN ART FORM AS WE USE IT TO HONOR AND NURTURE OURSELVES ON EVERY LEVEL. THE REJUV TOUCH RITUAL IS THE POINT WHERE TRANSFORMATION CAN TAKE PLACE, WHERE LETTING GO IS EASY, WHERE LIFE CAN BE RESTORED TO ITS NATURAL HARMONY, AND WHERE OUR UNIQUE BEAUTY IS REVEALED.

When we prepare both the inner and outer environments for the Daily Rejuv Touch Ritual, we provide the space and time to transform the emotional, mental, and behavioral qualities of our lives—the shapes and textures of the energies that flow to us, around us, and from us. With complete "presence" (conscious awareness), we use our hands to hold stillness at the nerve centers and to sweep along the pathways. By accessing our other levels through the nerve centers, we receive healing benefits and relaxation, body wide, at any time. With the Rejuv Breath, we connect to our core and reweave the integrity of the physical and energetic bodies.

The Daily Rejuv Touch Ritual is designed to hydrate, cleanse, and apply products. Its purpose is to treat the face and neck to a natural face-lift. The finest product we can use on our faces is our own tenderness. We will begin the Daily Rejuv Touch Ritual with "Soak to Save Your Face," a two-part process to hydrate and cleanse using the Press & Release technique. To apply products of your choice, we will continue with Pathways to Radiance, focusing on each area of the face and neck using the Finger Ripple and Sweep & Smooth techniques.

Our faces are the concrete expression of every pattern, every impact, every joy, and every trauma that we have experienced. The Daily Rejuv Touch Ritual helps dissolve multilevel crystallizations using various parts of the hands to release the micromuscle contractions. Reminding the cellular structures to expand, open, and uplift offers new, more flexible options of expression. When we decide to let go of feelings, thoughts, and actions that no longer serve us, we lighten our physiology and our spirits.

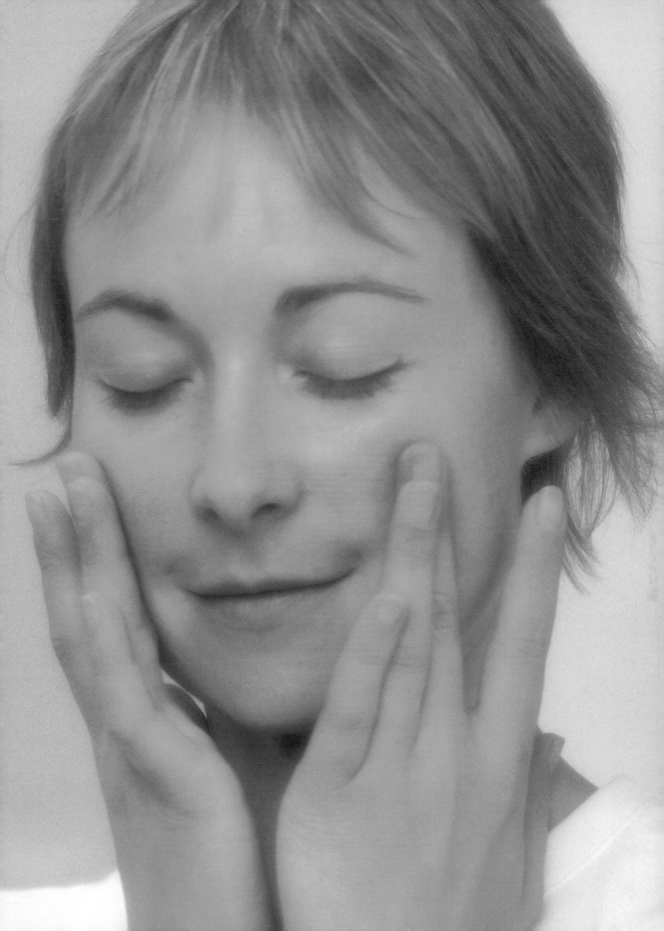

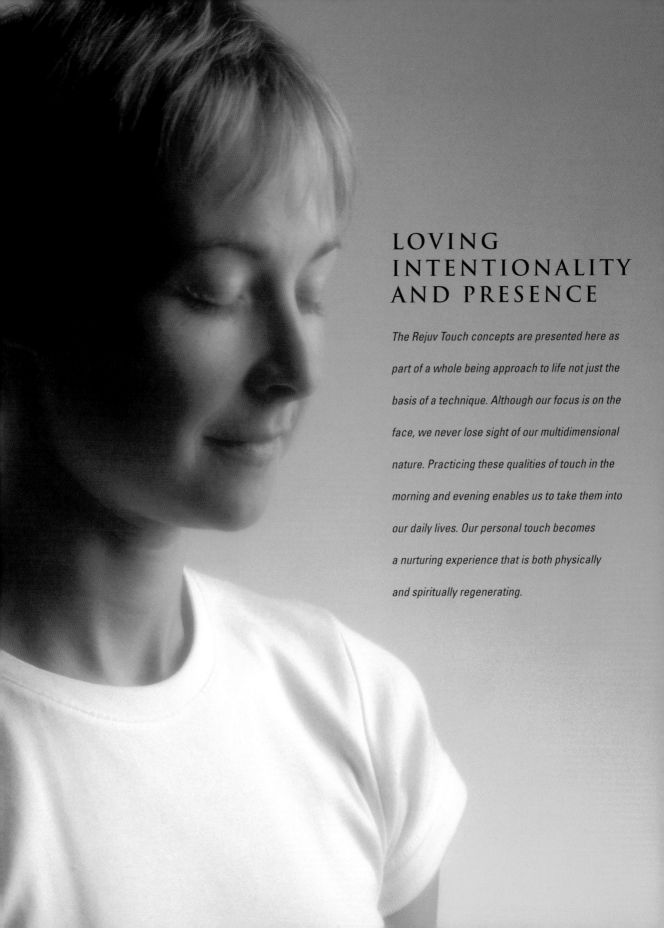

LOVING INTENTIONALITY AND PRESENCE

The Rejuv Touch concepts are presented here as part of a whole being approach to life not just the basis of a technique. Although our focus is on the face, we never lose sight of our multidimensional nature. Practicing these qualities of touch in the morning and evening enables us to take them into our daily lives. Our personal touch becomes a nurturing experience that is both physically and spiritually regenerating.

LOVING INTENTIONALITY

Love is a word we use all the time. We have a thousand different definitions and a thousand ways of loving. Perhaps one way in a thousand is based on unconditional loving. The rest often consist of manipulation and trade agreements—if I give you this, then I want that. If you give me that, what will I have to give? A simple act of love is not so simple when so many strings are attached. Yet, that one in a thousand—where love is unconditionally given and unconditionally received—that love has substance. It is the substance of love, a genuine physical substance that moves in, around, and through us all the time. It is life force. It is divine love. When you learn to perceive it, it feels as though you can rub it between your fingers. Loving intentionality is substantial; it can be generated; it can be sustained; and it can be felt.

This quality of love is an essential ingredient in the Rejuv Touch. We can hold the intention to be kind, to care, to nurture, to love unconditionally when we prepare to touch another, but often we do not bring these gifts to ourselves. We need to generate that same delightful, life-giving, joy-filled, sustaining love that we give to the special people in our lives whenever we prepare to do any self-care ritual.

PRESENCE

In order to touch with loving intentionality, we must be present. Presence is an illusive quality. You know when people have it and you know when they do not. We usually live within habitual patterns, often moving through daily routines on autopilot. If we pay closer attention to the sensory input we are receiving in each moment, the moment becomes alive and new. It is harder to notice subtle details when we are not present. Attention leads to awareness, which can give us more options—we can respond instead of react, we can communicate more effectively, we can engage fully with the world around us.

We want to move though our lives with the awareness that allows us to be present to whatever life offers us. The title of Ram Dass's book, *Be Here Now*, has become a catchphrase that is part of our culture and the global community. But how, though, can we really be more present? We begin with the densest aspect of who we are—the physical body. Gathering ourselves into this central core through the Rejuv Breath is one of the easiest ways to become present in any given moment. From this place we can establish connection with all our other levels. The body is our point of power. We start by being fully present in our hands and in our hearts for the rituals. We practice a few minutes a day—just with and for ourselves. From these precious moments, we develop the ability to stay present with ourselves, which allows us to have presence and be present with others in our lives.

REJUV BREATH MEDITATION—BOWL, HEART, AND HANDS

This meditation gives you a way to feel your own presence grounded in your own body. Begin using it in a quiet time and space, then you can use it anytime, even while standing, to reconnect to yourself quickly and deeply. This breath focuses your heart energies into your hands to make them tools for healing; these are your tools for the Rejuv Touch.

Sit or lie in a comfortable position. Close your eyes. See, feel, or imagine the air around you filled with sparkling golden energy—oxygen (physiological energy) and prana (light energy). Bring your breath and the sparkling energy through your nose and down into your body, into the bowl of your pelvis. This bowl is the pelvic girdle and includes winged hipbones, the pubic bone in front, and an arrow-shaped sacrum and tailbone in the back. It supports and cradles the root chakra, the spine, the nervous system, the internal organs, and the entire chakra system.

With each breath, the bowl fills with golden light until it overflows. Bring the overflow of sparkling golden energy up into your heart. With each breath, the overflow from the bowl rises to fill your heart until it also begins to overflow. Bring the heart's overflow of sparkling golden energy through your arms, and into your hands. Continue breathing the Rejuv Breath from nose to pelvis to heart to hands. Let your breath automatically follow this path, feeling grounded, centered, and connected. When you are ready, open your eyes, and have a good stretch.

We need to be nurtured to thrive. We know that as infants, our absolute survival depends not only on food and warmth but also on a loving human touch. As we grow, we learn to provide our own food and warmth and, although we do not outgrow our need for touch, we often neglect this aspect of our survival. All too often, we make ourselves dependent on others for a loving touch when, in fact, it can be self-generated.

A loving touch begins and ends with an awareness of the sacred, the life force that animates us, the essence of who we are. By dedicating time to these rituals on a daily basis, we tap into our own life force. The simple act of self-care is a nurturing moment: self-initiated, self-given, and self-accepted. Applying the Rejuv Touch principles is the key to awakening the body's innate wisdom and creating the spaciousness in our physical structures that allows us to expand in body, mind, and spirit.

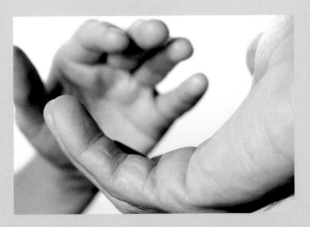

The Outer Setting—Creating Sacred Space

Although it can be helpful to have a dedicated area in our homes for sacred time, with clear intention we can create a sacred space within our own consciousness. This sacred space can be used anywhere and at any time. In the office, on a crowded street, in the middle of an argument, we can generate a sense of our own divine presence. We can reach into our own life-giving wholeness that is bigger than the location or the situation and that enfolds and touches the entire moment.

In our homes and bathrooms where most of the rituals take place, we can add all the little details to create a sacred space that is gracious and beautiful to all our senses. Before you begin a ritual, add a special candle, flowers, music, and scents that please you. Then settle undisturbed into this nurturing moment.

The Inner Setting—Accessing Sacred Space

Real and consistent inner connection can be difficult to maintain. However, daily practice in a controlled environment increases your ability to stay balanced in challenging situations. Using the Rejuv Drop (see below) allows you to enter into your core to create loving intentionality with and for yourself and to be fully present through whatever healing ritual you choose. The Daily Touch Ritual, practiced consistently for several weeks beginning with the Rejuv Drop, will change your relationship with yourself.

REJUV DROP MEDITATION

A quick and simple way to ground and connect to yourself is the Rejuv Drop. The Drop lowers your center of gravity physically, emotionally, and mentally. You can gather more of your multidimensional awareness into this grounded place, where "be here now" becomes effortless. First, practice feeling the weightedness of the drop in a quiet setting. Use it when you need to access the deeper inner strength and connection of presence.

1. To begin, simply bring your awareness to your shoulders. Let your shoulders drop into your hips, allowing your awareness and consciousness to drop with your shoulders. Feel your internal weight settle in your hips.

2. Once your shoulders have dropped and stabilized, drop your hips and shoulders to the floor. Let your whole sensory being join the drop. Feel your internal weight, awareness, and consciousness drop and stabilize.

3. When you feel stable, imagine that you can drop one level deeper, to the floor below or to the basement of your being. Again let all your weights drop. Stay at this depth as long as you can.

4. When you are ready, move into your day, breathing, acting, and speaking from the depth of your presence.

A touch can be a gift of both heart and hands. Touch is the primary way we learn about the world and is our first mode of communication. Learning the Rejuv Touch to improve our facial appearance may be the outward carrot. Truly to touch, though, we must begin an inward journey. We long to touch the truth of our hearts, our own inner connection to the divine, the beauty of our world, and the people we love. However haltingly or freely we touch, we must touch. But we also long to *be* touched—touched by the world around us, touched by the people we love, touched by the presence of God, touched by the light of the divine. The never-ending cycle of giving and receiving is what keeps us alive and engaged. Without touch some part of us begins to wither, so we touch and say *yes* to being touched, and the cycle keeps us going.

Conscious Slowness

Doing things slowly is not a normal state of affairs today, unless we are doing something we truly care about. In the Rejuv Touch, you will care deeply about what you are doing and will do it consciously. When you work slowly, you become aware of exactly what you are doing—what you are touching, how you are touching, where care is needed, when a cycle is complete. The sensory receptors in your hands can interact consciously with the sensory receptors being touched only if you work slowly.

This conscious slowness allows your physical systems—muscles, bones, blood, nerves, and lymph vessels—to reconnect with their energetic counterparts. Then both the physical and the energetic can nourish each other appropriately. When woven together, the two systems are recharged, cleansed, and integrated. Give yourself permission to work slowly, with presence, feeling the structures beneath your hands completely. Working slowly seems to stretch time because your senses come alive to what you are actually touching. Following the contours of bones, muscles, and skin becomes a journey of awareness and attentiveness.

These timeless moments of self care carried out with conscious slowness are more effective and more satisfying than rushing through a routine.

Holding in Stillness

Moments of stillness, when we simply hold with presence and loving intentionality, are as important as moments of movement. When we hold, we allow integration. It is in the stillness that we can accept, receive, and integrate what is moving in flows of energy. When you reach a nerve center, hold it in stillness.

Beginning, Middle, and End

There is a sequence to all things—to a ritual, to a sweep, to a single touch—and each stage moves smoothly into the next. An awareness of where you begin, where you end, and the journey between the two creates a continuous connective experience. Each touch, sweep, and moment of stillness is important because a release can occur anywhere.

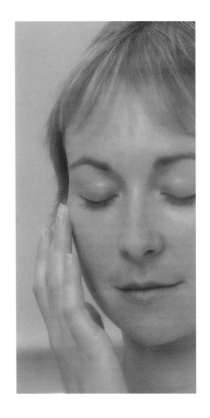

Whether your primary interest is in the physical condition of your face or a greater experience of vitality in your life, the Rejuv Rituals throughout this book offer a point of entry for you. Dissolving and releasing our emotional crystallizations is an integral part of the Rejuv Touch. These crystallizations (emotional patterns held in the cells) and their micromuscle contractions within your face impede the free flow of energy, blood, and nourishment. They are sustained by outdated thoughts, feelings, and behaviors. Releasing the old to make way for the new is a core transformational concept. Release can happen in many ways. In Rejuv, we rely on the interconnectedness of our multilevel system. We use the Rejuv pathways and the nerve centers on the face and neck to release bound energy body-wide.

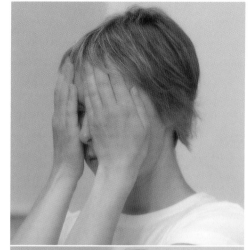

In each moment, with each ritual, we simply offer ourselves the grace of our own loving. Emotional crystallizations can effortlessly dissolve and enter the flow again. We have committed on some level to reach for wholeness and these rituals offer the possibility of letting go of what stands in the way. This can be a conscious process—a simple touch may trigger a memory to release. It may be an other-than-conscious process—a deep breath may signal a deep release of some forgotten injury. We may never know which thoughts and feelings have taken the physical form of emotional crystallizations in our cells; we do not need to know. We only need to remind these cells, through silent and loving cellular communication, that they can return to their original state of relaxation, of health, of beauty—ultimate wholeness.

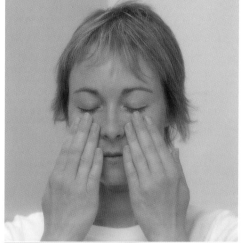

When you are doing the Press & Release, the Finger Ripple, and the Sweep & Smooth, be inspired as you communicate with your cells. You can speak in physical terms ("All the toxins in the cells are free to leave my body"), emotional terms ("I forgive myself for holding on to these negative feelings"), mental terms ("I can release all thoughts of lack and contraction"), and spiritual terms ("My divine expression radiates from all my cells"). With ongoing cellular communication, there will be a shift in perception—which is one definition of a miracle.

Through daily repetition of the Rejuv Touch Ritual, the nerve centers will be activated and synchronized, and the Rejuv pathways will be cleared and refreshed. Bound energy dissolved from crystallizations and micromuscle contractions will begin to flow freely. As you become more familiar with the process, you will feel different levels of energy and release throughout your body. Your facial muscles, released from the tension of old holding patterns, will reflect your unique beauty, unobstructed by past trauma. Your true essence will become more and more visible.

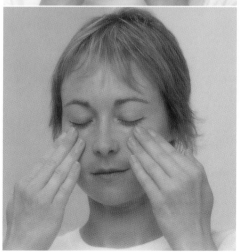

The opposite of closed is open. The opposite of contraction is expansion. The opposite of downward is upward. There is a time for closing, contracting, and moving in downward flows, just as there is a time for opening, expanding, and lifting into upward flows. It is the dance of balance between these opposites that allows our bodies to sustain themselves and that permits life to move forward.

The focus of the Rejuv Touch is to help reverse the tendency to close and contract instead of opening and expanding to whatever life brings us. The purpose of all the positions, sweeps, and holds is to expand, uplift, and open contractions on all levels. In this technique, movement is always from the center of the face (midline) to the outside (coronal) with a slight upward intention (Lift to Smile). The Daily Touch Ritual impacts the musculature of the face by shifting it into lift, not sag.

The specific patterns in Press & Release, Finger Ripple, and Sweep & Smooth enliven and strengthen the energetic and physical structures of regeneration and rejuvenation. A gentle sweep along the Rejuv pathways activates the energetic and physical flows, and a tender hold at each nerve center awakens and synchronizes them. These sequences naturally begin to uplift, open, and expand all the areas of the face.

As you prepare to begin the work, be aware that there are no throwaway moments. Whether you dedicate an hour to do some of the longer rituals or spend three minutes soaking your face, make the time conscious, deliberate, and connected. Every moment of stillness and every movement can enhance, refresh, and uplift your multidimensional radiance.

The intention throughout the process, whether you are doing a Press & Release, Finger Ripple, or Sweep & Smooth, is your deep connection with the bones of the face. The energy of this bone-to-bone (hands on face) connection passes through and affects all the cells—skin, muscle, blood, lymph, nerves, and the connective tissue in between. You maintain full contact with as little muscular distortion as possible, neither pushing nor pulling the skin.

Lift to Smile

The intention of Lift to Smile is to place the corners of a tiny smile at each nerve center. You will hold an angle of lift in stillness each time you touch a nerve center. This is a 45-degree angle between the midline and the coronal plane, not up to the ceiling nor out to the sides, but in between, like the grin of the Cheshire cat. The skin will move slightly in the direction of the lift, but it is your intention that does the job of uplifting and expanding, not the physical pull. Your physical effort is so gentle that the skin moves within the intention of the lift. The Lift to Smile will not create stretch damage to the delicate facial tissue. Your focus is lightly physical but mostly energetic, and your intention implants the memory of a joyous, easy, lighter response to life.

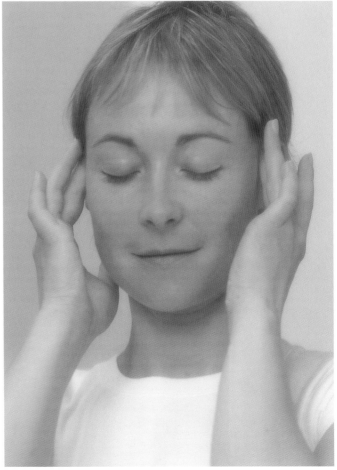

YOUR HEALING HANDS

Slicing a carrot, holding a glass, threading a needle, turning a screw, caressing a loved one, wiping a tear—our hands perform each of these simple actions without hesitation. While constantly in motion, our hands are the tools of daily life and daily loving. Our hands shape the world around us and make manifest both the dreams and the necessities of our lives.

Hands are delicate, strong, and flexible. So much life encompassed in this complex rigging of bones, sinew, muscles, and nerves. Through the Rejuv Breath Meditation, we will connect to the flow of life force coursing through the physical body, strengthening the communication from heart to fingertips, and our hands will become healing instruments.

Begin by being fully aware of your hands as you apply the Rejuv Touch. Whether you are using your whole palm or a single finger pad, touch with full presence. This level of presence carries its own weight, and there is no need for added physical pressure. The following exercise will give you the quality of the Rejuv Touch you will use for all the rituals.

PRESENCE NOT PRESSURE EXERCISE

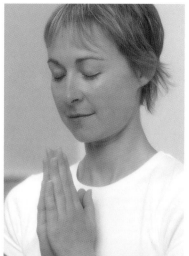

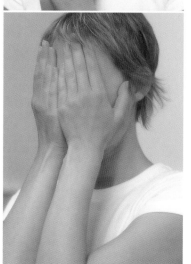

Settle yourself into the bowl of the pelvis (Rejuv Breath) and bring your hands together in a loose prayer position—heels touch, then palms, then fingers. Notice how your hands feel as they rest against each other.

Keeping your hands together, relax into your breath and close your eyes. Begin to see, feel, or imagine your hands melting into each other, as though the bones of one hand were melting into the bones of the other.

Starting with the little fingers, melt long bones into long bones, knuckles into knuckles; at the joints, creases of skin open and melt into each other and at the tips, pads melt into one another. Next, your ring finger bones melt, knuckles merging, skin creases, and tips merging. Then your middle fingers melt—bones, knuckles, creases, fingertips—followed by your index fingers melting one into the other. Last, the entire length of your thumbs, from heels to tips, melts one into the other. Breathe deeply; feel yourself centered in your hands.

Now focus on the very center of your palms, and allow the bones of your palms to melt into one other. The space between your palms diminishes until you no longer feel any space between them. Focus your breath into your palms.

Feel your presence in each hand as they connect deeply with each other. Allow energy to travel between your hands—left hand melting into right, then right melting into left. Continue the gentle movement of your full presence between your hands.

Slowly, peel your hands away from each other—heels, palms, then fingers—while retaining the memory of the melt. Gently place your hands on your face, letting the bones of your hands melt into the bones beneath your touch. Be present—bone to bone, muscle to muscle, skin to skin—and allow the energy to flow from the pelvis to the heart and hands and into the face. With this flow of energy, focus on loving intentionality, cellular communication, releasing, and uplifting. Softly and gently peel your hands from your face and let them rest in your lap. Experience the quality of the touch you have created in your hands, on your face, and in your whole body. This is presence.

HAND POSITIONS

Begin each ritual with the Rejuv Breath and the Presence exercise to dedicate your hands as nurturing instruments. Bring your full presence to each part of your hands as you touch. Imagine your hands moving through the viscosity of thick, warm honey; slowly they reach your face, sweep to a nerve center then hold in stillness. Each ritual can be just another technique or a healing experience; the difference is in your awareness.

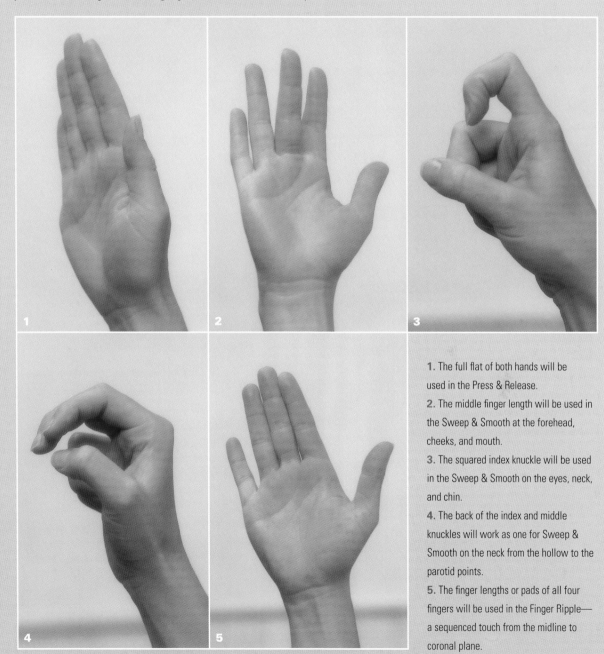

1. The full flat of both hands will be used in the Press & Release.

2. The middle finger length will be used in the Sweep & Smooth at the forehead, cheeks, and mouth.

3. The squared index knuckle will be used in the Sweep & Smooth on the eyes, neck, and chin.

4. The back of the index and middle knuckles will work as one for Sweep & Smooth on the neck from the hollow to the parotid points.

5. The finger lengths or pads of all four fingers will be used in the Finger Ripple— a sequenced touch from the midline to coronal plane.

We've journeyed through our stories and nutritional guidelines, located the nerve centers and pathways, and explored the Rejuv concepts. The Daily Rejuv Touch Ritual puts it all together. Used as part of your morning and evening routine, the Rejuv Touch Ritual will greatly enhance the texture of your skin, refine your pores, and increase circulation. We begin with Soak to Save Your Face—hydration and cleansing—using the Press & Release. We end with Pathways to Radiance. Different parts of the hands will focus on each area of the face doing continual, smoothing sweeps along the pathways. Products are applied with the Finger Ripple and Sweep & Smooth. Without products, and only your loving attention, you can reweave your physical and energetic structures allowing your radiance to freely come forward.

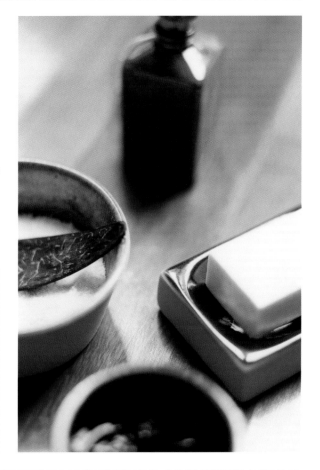

PRODUCTS

• Your favorite facial cleanser, toner, moisturizer, and essential oils.

• The best products contain high-quality organic ingredients with little or no processing and no chemical additives, preservatives, or coloring agents—remember good, better, best (Chapter 2).

• If you would not want to eat it, do not put it on your face.

REJUV PATHWAYS REVIEW

FOREHEAD: From the midline arching across the frontal bones to the temple points.

EYES: From the bridge of the nose, outline the curve of the eye to the temple point. Upper eye: On the edge of the riser of the orbital bone. Lower eye: On the edge of the riser on the top of the cheekbone.

CHEEKS: From the bridge of the nose across the wide expanse of the tread of the cheekbone to the triangle ear points, directly across to the ears, not following the downward curve of the cheekbone.

MOUTH: From the center of the lips to the mouth corner points, Lift to Smile, then trace across the spongy, hollow cheek area to the triangle ear points.

CHIN: From the cleft, along the tread, the riser or the edge of the jawbone, around the ramus and up to the parotids.

NECK: First up from the hollow to the jawbone, then along the edge of the riser of the jawbone, around the ramus, and up to the parotids, opening the fan in three channels. Complete one side, then do the other, using opposite hands.

PRESS & RELEASE

We will use the Press & Release for the hydration and cleansing rituals and to remove facial masks (Chapter 6). Both hydration and cleansing rituals are performed bending over a bathroom basin or bowl with your face above the water. In this position, gravity helps the lymph to move and flow, draining excessive fluids from the tissues of the face and neck, especially the eyelids, cheeks, and jowls. Use either full hands holding a washcloth or the long lengths of your fingers to mold around the contours of your face, sinking into its bony structure.

Press & Release focuses on a bone-to-bone connection. As you press, your hand connects fully with the facial bones. There is full cellular communication and energetic exchange with complete presence but no push. The gentle press increases blood and lymph circulation and stimulates nerve function, which is essential to healthy, glowing skin. It allows emotional and energetic crystallizations in the cells to be loosened and released so that they are free to flow into the pathways and nerve centers.

Facial muscles, even the smallest micromuscles, that are locked in a habitual range of motion or position can be pressed and released. As they regain elasticity, they can move beyond habit into new expressions. Once these micromuscles receive a fresh nutrient supply from the stimulated blood flow, they are able to support the emotional and energetic shifts. The outgoing toxins, carried away by the lymph, leave space for nourishment and nutrients. The cellular structures receiving the raw material can generate healthy new cells that are not as locked into the old emotional and physical holding patterns. By doing the Press & Release mornings and evening, the skin's efficiency of function and your facial expressions will both receive a daily renewal.

How to Press & Release

1. Both hands press simultaneously: full hands with washcloth or full length of fingers to apply cleanser.

2 a–b. Full hands cover forehead, eyes, and cheeks. Press & Release gently from the midline to the coronal plane.

3 a–c. Lower the hands to cover eyes, nose, cheeks, mouth, and chin. Press & Release gently from the midline to the coronal plane.

4. End Press & Release sequence with opposite hands on the neck.

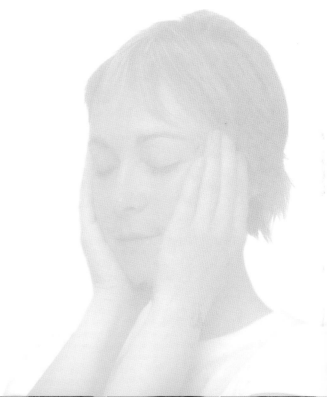

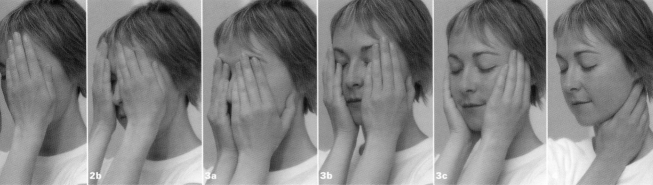

SOAK TO SAVE YOUR FACE

The skin's aging process is not a matter of loss of oil as much as it is due to loss of water. It is a myth of the cosmetic industry that an oil-rich (and very expensive) cream will hydrate your skin cells. In truth, the simplicity of a morning and evening soak with warm water will hydrate all the layers of your skin, thus activating the natural regeneration process. Consistent hydration is the key to bringing the skin back to efficient functioning.

A good facial soak is like a tiny bath and produces results similar to a whole body bath. The wet warmth from your face transmits relaxation throughout your body as it soothes your nervous system. You may not have the time for a bath, but you can always find the time (less than three minutes) for this deep soak.

When you wash your face while standing in the shower, you fail to use the natural force of gravity to assist the lymphatic flow in your face and neck. Leaning over a bowl or the bathroom basin, however, allows gravity to pull debris, toxins, and residues from deep facial tissue layers. We recognize our internal need for water, but the body's outer need for hydration is also essential. Beyond cleanliness, water also assists exfoliation by softening the epidermal surface of the skin and enhances the immune system by detoxifying through the pores. The heated moisture of the cloth opens pores and softens and exfoliates dead skin cells to be gently rinsed away. Once your face is hydrated, cleanser, toner, moisturizer, and makeup will all be more effective.

HYDRATION RITUAL

1. Fill a bowl or bathroom basin with hot water that is just comfortable to the touch.

2. Add three to six drops of essential oil, floral water, hydro-sol or Jurlique Aromatic Hydrating Concentrate (see Resources) to the water.

3. Lean your face over the water and remain in this position throughout the process (you may rest your elbows on the counter for support).

4. Soak your washcloth in the hot, fragrant water, and bring the wet cloth to your face.

5. Beginning at the midline, press the cloth into the skin and hold for a few moments; communicate.

6. Press & Release again, moving hands slightly outward and following the pathways toward the coronal plane. Each press covers large portions of a pathway, ending with a press at a nerve center.

7. As you reach each nerve center, pause and hold. Resoak the cloth to reheat and move to the midline again, positioning hands slightly lower. Work from your forehead to your neck.

8. At the neck, gently use the opposite hand to do the Press & Release from the hollow to the parotids.

9. Allow heat, water, fragrance, and intention to soak into the layers of your skin.

10. As the cloth cools, release and resoak. While leaning over, continue the Press & Release.

11. Repeat press (communicate) and release (resoak) over your entire face and neck, eight to ten times.

12. Dry your hands slightly, leaving the face and neck moist to continue with the cleansing ritual.

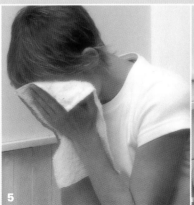
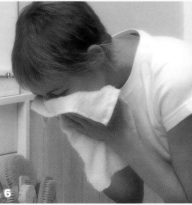
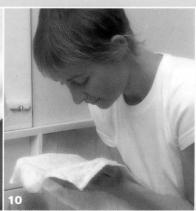

CLEANSING RITUAL

When we were children, our mothers often scrubbed our faces clean. Scrubbing did get the dirt off, but this method also shoved and stretched the skin randomly, crumpling the tissue and bunching the energy fields. While scrubbing may have served its purpose at the time, it is certainly not conducive to the refinement of tissue and bony structure that we seek as adults. Scrubbing the face does not support synchronization of the physical and energetic structures.

Using the Press & Release technique to cleanse the skin will refresh the free and active flows of the Rejuv pathways. This cleansing method actively supports detoxification from the pores, moving the skin toward more efficient function. The deliberate press stimulates the deeper layers of skin cells to loosen toxins and the dead skin cells to exfoliate. The release allows gravity to pull toxins and debris gently to the surface layers to be removed with the cleanser without scrubbing.

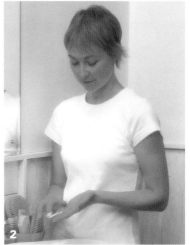

To Apply:

1. Apply a small amount of cleanser to the palm of your hand, add a little hot water, and blend together.

2. Cover finger lengths of both hands with the mixture.

3. Lean over the sink. Press the cleanser onto your face along the Rejuv pathways with infinite tenderness. Communicate.

4. Beginning at the midline, press the cleanser into the skin, and hold for a count of three; communicate.

5. Continue to release and press, each time moving hands slightly outward, following the pathways toward a nerve center.

6. Return to the midline after each nerve center has been held.

7. Reapply cleanser to fingers as needed as you press and release from your forehead to your neck.

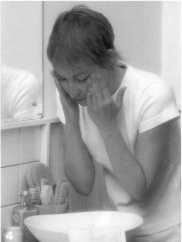

To Remove:

8. Resoak the washcloth used in the Hydration Ritual in warm water.

9. Repeat the same pattern as the Hydration Ritual, gently pressing the water into the skin to loosen the cleanser and releasing to resoak the cloth.

10. Press and release until all the cleanser is removed.

11. To end, rinse the cloth in cool water for one last press and release.

Optional Ending:

12. Wrap the cloth around your hand to create a mitt. Sweep & Smooth along the Rejuv pathways to a nerve center, treating first one side, then the other.

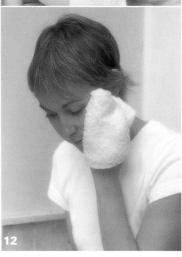

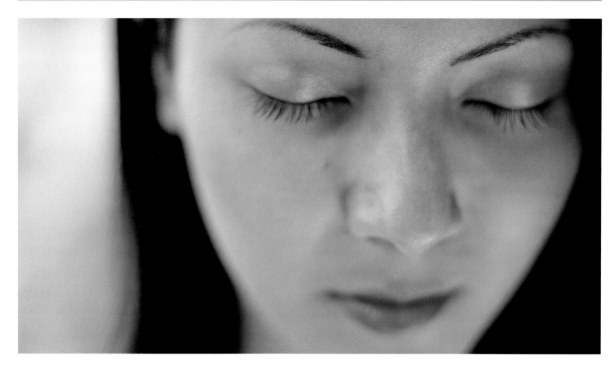

Application Ritual: Sweep & Smooth

This ritual is designed to apply products to the face and neck to create a natural face-lift. The Sweep & Smooth treatment in each area will differ slightly. The intention of the sweep is to stimulate, clear, cleanse, and refresh the Rejuv pathways and bring new radiance to the physical and energetic structures of the face and neck.

The application ritual is simple but requires a shift from the unconscious, get-it-done-quickly application habits we have been doing each morning. This self-care ritual requires consciousness and presence. Using presence in the Rejuv Touch creates full contact, energetically connecting all our levels and synchronizing their flows and functions. The Sweep & Smooth sequence refines bony structure, tones facial muscles, and synchronizes nerve communication—benefits well worth the learning of new habits and behaviors.

We suggest you use the sweeps not only to apply your favorite products but also to apply tenderness and love to each area of your face. When performed gently on bare skin, these sweeps can renew the energetic flows of the body, mind, and emotions. You may do them individually or in the series as described below. In a short time, you will begin to feel body-wide refreshment. Since the shapes of faces and hands vary widely, the instructions in the application ritual will give you only a general map of placement. Follow the map as best you can, shifting fingers and knuckles to fit the unique contours of your face and hands.

The Sweep & Smooth is one continuous movement of your fingers or knuckles from the midline to a nerve center. There are no stops and starts, no lifting off or pushing back, just a smooth continuous flow expanding toward the coronal plane and lifting at the nerve center. You work with presence, and a conscious intention of bone-to-bone cellular communication, not pressure. The skin will move slightly over the bones, but with presence—not pressure—the cellular structure will not stretch into distortion but lift into alignment. Strengthening and connecting the energy flows with the Sweep & Smooth on a daily basis (with or without facial products) will begin to restore elasticity to the soft tissue, resiliency to the bones, and a natural glow to the skin.

Products are initially applied with the Finger Ripple. Then the Sweep & Smooth is used to spread the product evenly over the face. For each area the procedure will be shown separately.

FINGER RIPPLE

This technique blends aspects of the Press & Release with the Sweep & Smooth. The combined actions release micromuscle holding patterns and immediately move the loosened energy toward a nerve center to be reintegrated or released from your system. Continue to focus on the cellular communication from the bones of your fingers to the bones of your face.

The Finger Ripple is a wavelike sequence using full flat fingers or pads to Press & Release within the continual flow of a Sweep & Smooth. The ring, middle, and index fingers press in sequence on a single Rejuv pathway beginning at the midline. Then, as a unit, the fingers lift off the skin slightly, move outward toward the coronal plane, and return to another sequenced press, eventually ending at a nerve center.

The Finger Ripple is an ideal technique for the initial application of any product (toner, moisturizer, foundation, masks, suntan lotion) to the face. It can be followed by the Sweep & Smooth to spread the product evenly on each area.

Use the Finger Ripple to apply products to the entire face and neck *before* performing the Sweep & Smooth on each area.

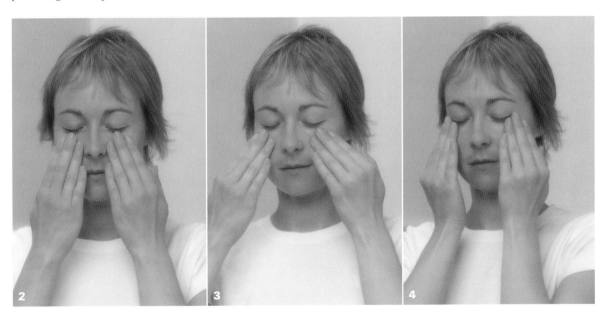

1. Apply a small amount of product to the pads or full lengths of your fingers, depending on the size of the area to be covered and the size of your hands.

2. Ring, middle, and index fingers are placed as a unit on the face, ring finger at the midline.

3. With infinite tenderness, each finger will press deeper into the tissue in sequence—first the ring finger, then the middle finger, and then the index finger. Communicate as you press.

4. As a unit, the three fingers lift barely off the skin to move slightly outward, following the pathways toward the designated nerve center.

5. Repeat the ripple: place fingers, press-press-press, lift, move.

6. Repeat until the ring finger presses at a nerve center.

7. At the next pathway, return to the midline and repeat the Finger Ripple to its nerve center at the coronal plane.

8. Reapply product to fingers as needed and continue the Finger Ripple until finished.

FOREHEAD

Your own touch of love and self-care is infused into each product you use. The application of this touch is the true intention that renews the pathways to radiance for you. The application of product is to focus your attention in an easy way to include the Rejuv Touch in your daily routine. Remember, you can also do the sweeps alone at any time.

The wide pathway of the forehead covers a broad expanse of the frontal bone on the tread: from brows to hairline and from midline to temples. The flow within this pathway begins at the midline between the brows, arches up the midline toward the hairline, and opens below the hairline following the arch to each temple point.

1. Apply product as needed to the full length of fingers. Smooth with the full length of middle finger, spreading the liquid across the forehead, using no pressure, just presence and deliberate intention.

2. To begin the Sweep & Smooth, place your middle finger pads at the midline between the brows.

3. Staying in full contact sweep up the midline.

4. With deliberate slowness sweep up to the hairline.

5. Remaining just below the hairline, open outwards following the contour of the forehead.

6. Follow the arching of the hairline to the coronal plane, toward the temples.

7. At the temple point, hold for three counts.

8. Lift to Smile, and hold for another count of three.

9. Repeat the sweep two more times.

10. At the end of the third sweep, touch the pituitary point, then touch the crown point (see page 75, # 6a–c).

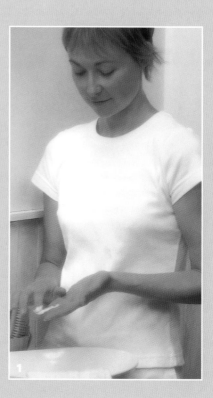

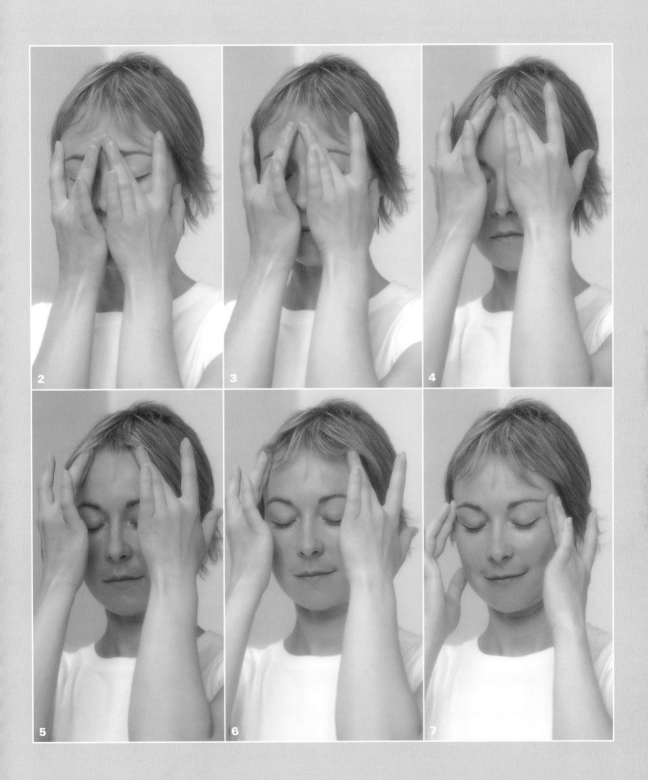

As we approach the eyes, we do so with added care, tenderness, and awareness. Deliberate slowness and presence are even more important in this area. We do not want to stretch the skin around the eyes, but we do want to refresh the pathways actively and move crystallizations through the area.

The eyes have both an upper and a lower pathway. Each pathway follows the contour of the bony orbital ridge on the edge of the riser surrounding each eye. The upper pathway flows from just above the inner corner of the eye (inner canthus), following the upper arch to the outer corner (outer canthus), and ending at the temple point. The lower pathway flows from just below the inner canthus, following the lower arch to the outer canthus, and ending at the temple point.

Upper Eye

The upper eye Sweep & Smooth allows the musculature of the brow and eye tissue to be relaxed and redefined.

1. Apply a small amount of product to your index finger knuckles.
2. Rest the flat of the knuckles near the bridge of your nose.
3. Sweep along the edge of the riser, following the curve of the upper orbital bone to the outer corner of the eyes.

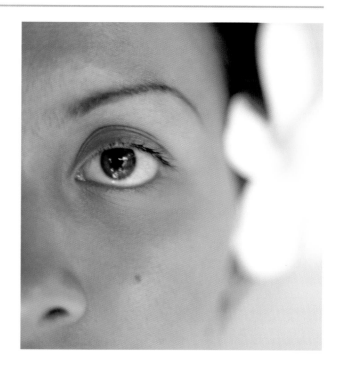

4. Trace the squared knuckles to the temple point and hold for three counts.
5. At the temple point, Lift to Smile, and hold for another count of three.
6. Repeat the sweep twice more.
7. At the end of the third sweep, touch the pituitary, then touch the crown (see page 75, # 6 a–c).

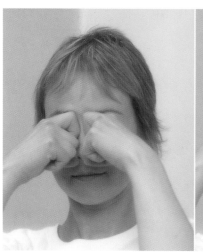
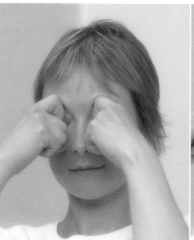
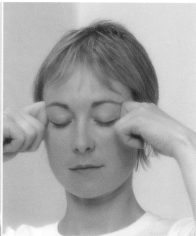

Lower Eye

The lower eye Sweep & Smooth begins to uplift the flows and expand the musculature in the cheeks as well as in the eye tissue.

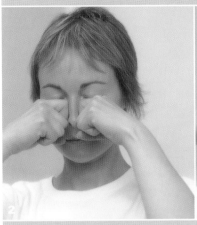 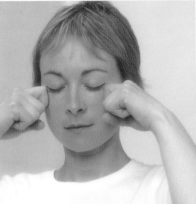 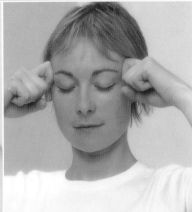

1. Apply a small amount of product to your squared index finger knuckles.

2. Rest the flats of the knuckles near the bridge of your nose.

3. Sweep along on the edge of the tread of the upper cheekbone to the outer corner of the eyes.

4. Trace the knuckle tips to the temple point and hold for three counts.

5 a–c. At the temple point, Lift to Smile, and hold for another count of three.

6. Repeat the sweep two more times. At the end of the third sweep, touch the pituitary, then touch the crown (see page 75, # 6 a–c).

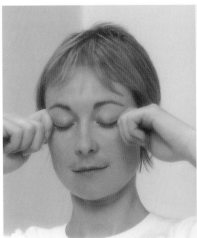 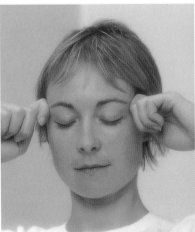 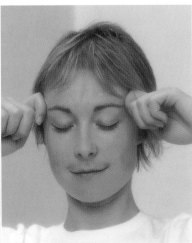

CHEEKS

When you use Sweep & Smooth on the cheeks, it is essential to focus on widening the bony structure and uplifting the skin tissue. The pathway flows from the midline on the bridge of the nose, out along the flat of the cheekbones, to the triangle ear points. Use the flat surface of the bone to guide the expansion and lifting. If you follow the downward shape of the lower cheekbone, you will add to the gravity of the area and cause the tissue to sag rather than to be uplifted.

This wide pathway covers the broad expanse of the cheeks on the tread: from the bridge of the nose to the coronal plane and from just below the edge of the lower orbital ridge to the edge of the tread of the lower cheekbone. The flow within this pathway has several channels, all of which begin at the midline and continue down the sides of the nose, across the cheeks, and ending at either the triangle ear points or with a slight curve to the temples (depending on the ritual).

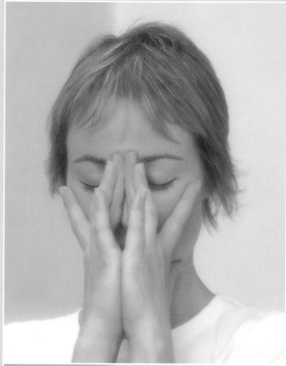

1. Apply product as needed to the flat finger lengths.

2. Place the middle fingers full-length together along the midline on the bridge of the nose.

3. Sweep gently down the sides of the nose.

4. With deliberate slowness, sweep across the wide expanse of the cheek area.

5. Follow the contours of the cheek lifting slightly toward the ears.

6. Slide fingertips to triangle ear points, hold for a count of three.

7. Lift to Smile and hold for another count of three.

8. Repeat the sweep two more times.

9. At the end of the third sweep, touch the pituitary, then touch the crown (see page 75, # 6 a–c).

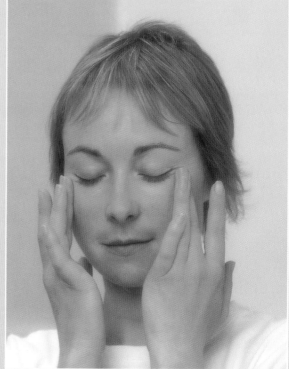

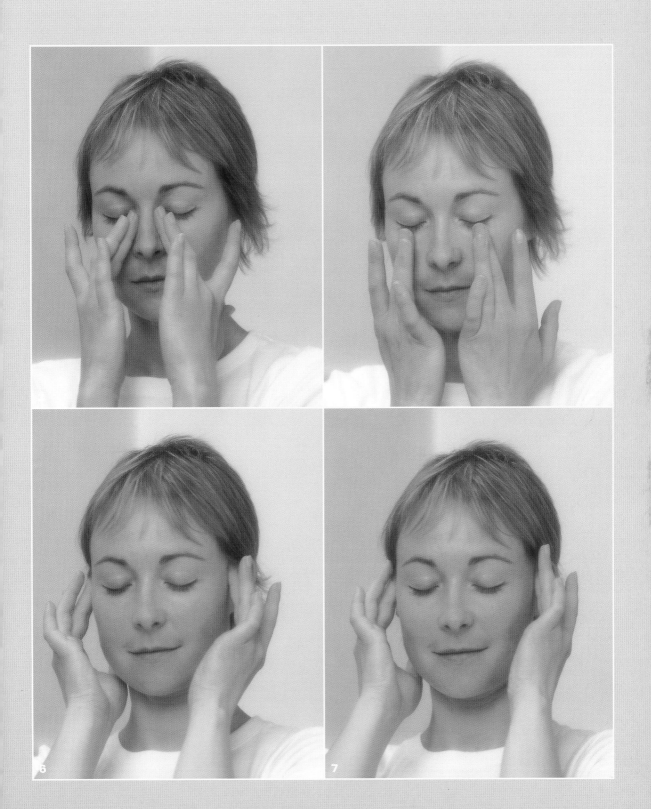

MOUTH

Performing the Sweep & Smooth on the mouth requires both
delicacy and presence. You want to encourage the corners of your
lips to curve upward in a smile. Your goal is to nudge the
micromuscle contractions toward an open smile with no
distortion of the musculature and skin. This Lift to Smile at the
mouth corner points is more visible but as small as at all the
other nerve centers.

FIRST FLOW

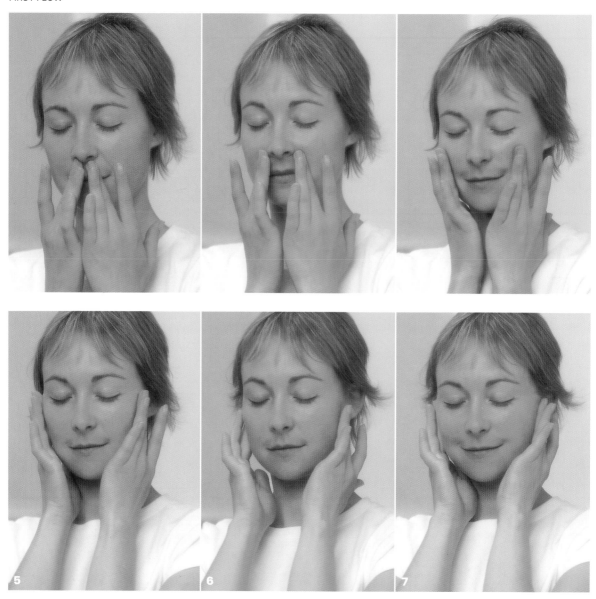

This complete pathway encompasses the area below the cheeks and nose down to the jawbone from the midline to the coronal plane. There are two distinct flows in this pathway; first from midline directly to parotid points, second from midline to mouth corner points and, from mouth corner points to parotid points.

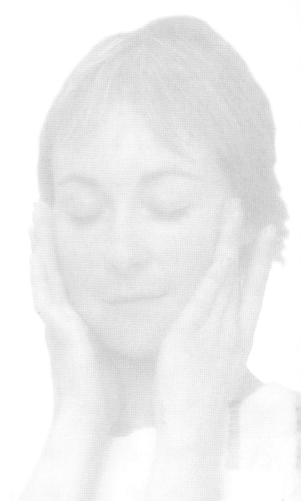

First Flow

1. Apply product to the fingers as needed as you cover the area—from lower cheekbones to jawline; from lips to triangle ear points.

2. Place the middle fingers across the lips, from nose to chin.

3. Sweep gently over the mouth corner points.

4. Smooth across the hollow of the cheek area with full presence.

5. Follow the contours of the cheeks out toward the coronal plane.

6. Slide the fingertips to the triangular ear points and hold for a count of three.

7. Lift to Smile and hold for another count of three.

8. Apply product as needed. Repeat steps 2–7 for two more sweeps.

Second Flow

9. Place your middle finger pads on both lips at the midline.

10. Sweep gently to the mouth corner points. Hold for three counts.

11. Lift to Smile and hold for another count of three.

12. To complete this second flow, repeat steps 4–6.

13. Repeat this sequence two more times.

14. At the end of the third sweep, touch the pituitary point, then touch the crown point (see page 75, # 6a–c).

SECOND FLOW

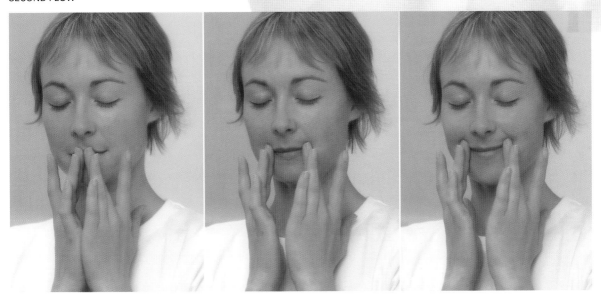

NECK

In sweeping and smoothing the neck, we are creating a shape that resembles the opening of a fan. At the midline the fan is closed. With each successive sweep up a new channel, the fan opens wider until the fan is fully opened and expanded at the parotids. You can perform the full opening once or repeat it a few times.

This pathway is shaped like an open fan, with the handle of the fan resting in the hollow and opening to each of the parotid points. The energy flow within this pathway covers two areas—the tread of the neck and the riser of the chin and jaw—in multiple channels. Within these channels, the flows begin at the hollow and follow the contours of the neck and chin to the edge of the tread of the jawbone. They end either by flowing along this edge to the parotid points or into the energy field at the jawbone.

KEY

■ Neck pathway

→ First channel

→ Second channel

→ Third channel

FIRST CHANNEL

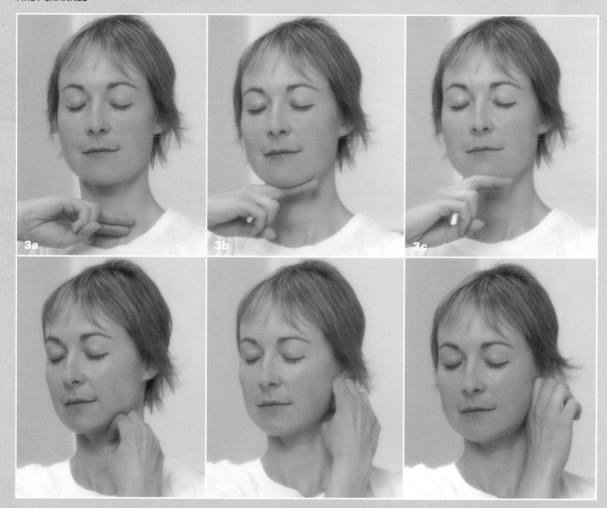

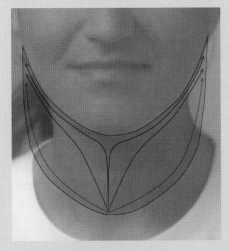

1. Apply the product to back of the middle knuckles (index and middle fingers). Use the right hand for the left side, then the left hand for the right side.

2. Place the flats of the index and middle finger knuckles at the hollow to begin sweeping each of the three channels opening approximately 1 inch (2.5 cm) with every stroke.

3 a–f. First channel: up the midline from the hollow to the chin, sweep along the edge of the jawbone, around the ramus, and up to the parotid point; hold for a count of three; then Lift to Smile and hold for another count of three.

4 a–c. Second channel: up from the hollow to the jaw, open the fan and sweep along the edge of the jawbone, around the ramus, and up to the parotid point; hold for a count of three, then Lift to Smile and hold for another count of three.

5 a–c. Third channel: sweep up from the hollow directly to the parotid point; hold for a count of three, then Lift to Smile and hold for another count of three.

6. Repeat the procedure on the other side.

SECOND CHANNEL

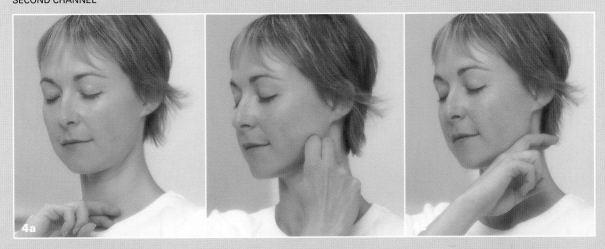

THIRD CHANNEL

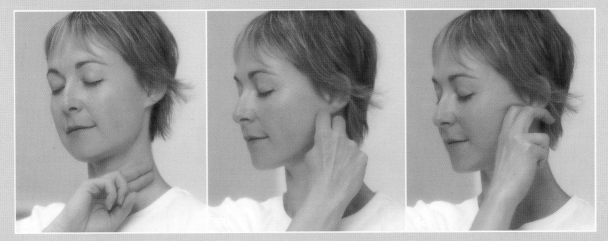

CHIN

In this final Sweep & Smooth, we will focus our attention on opening and expanding the chin the major reflex area for the pelvic girdle. The neck work included sweeps along the tread of the jawbone and began movement of energy in the chin pathway. Your touch, as you travel along the pathway, is light and conscious. With deliberate slowness, you will feel all the nooks and crannies of the edge of the chin and jawbone, and only slightly disturb the musculature and skin.

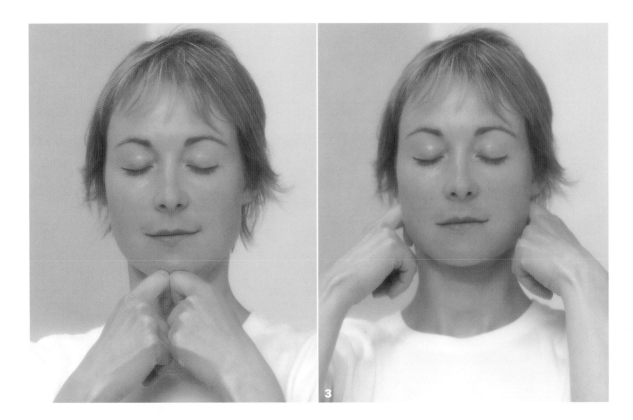

The pathway of the chin follows the jawbone from the cleft of the chin to the parotid points. The flow moves within the whole bone—tread, riser, and the edge in between.

1. Apply the product to the back of the index finger knuckles.

2. Place your squared knuckles on the tip of your chin.

3. Sweep along the edge of the jaw, around the ramus, and up to the parotid points, then hold for three counts.

4. Lift to Smile and hold for another count of three.

5. Repeat the sweep two more times.

6 a–c. At the end of the third sweep, touch the pituitary point, then touch the crown point.

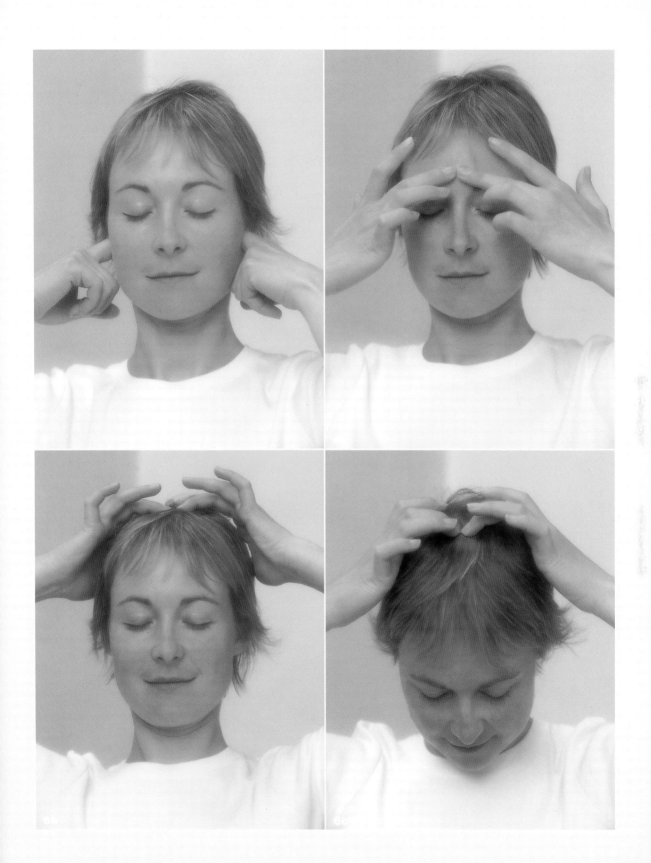

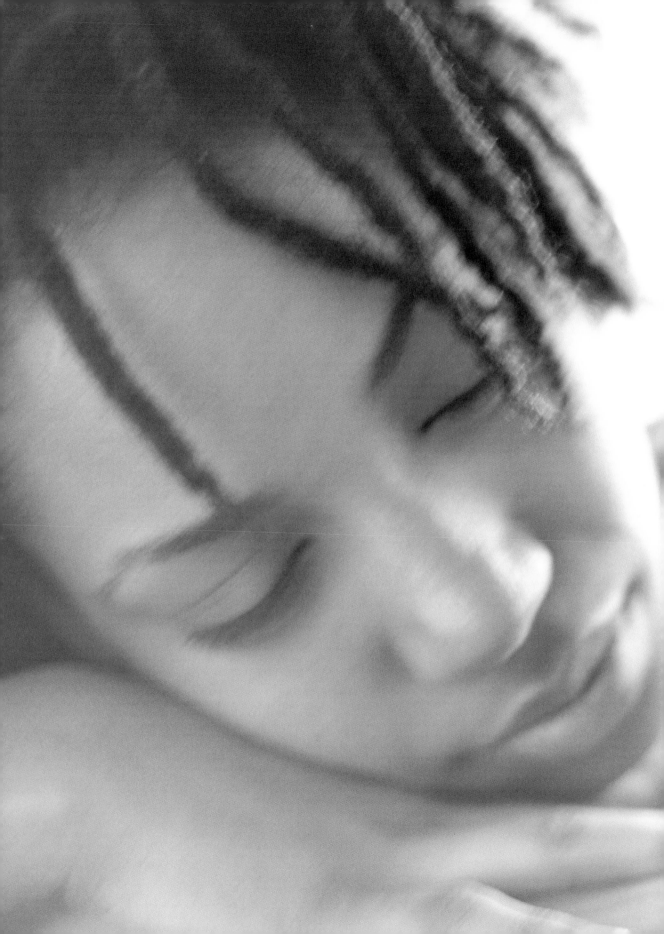

PART TWO:

SELF-CARE
RITUALS

The self-care rituals in Part Two will shift your focus from hygiene to nourishment and renewal. These practical and simple rituals will not focus on the skin and face alone since true beauty is not just skin-deep. Beauty comes from wholeness. Therefore, we offer you rituals, routines, and suggestions that will lead to a full-body regeneration and rejuvenation.

These rituals refocus your attention from simple physical self-care to a deeper consideration of all your needs: rituals for your face and body, new ways of nurturing your energy flow, quick methods for relaxing your feelings and emotions, and a gentle touch for bringing peace and clarity to your entire being. Step-by-step instructions and illustrations combine beauty routines with natural products, visualizations and meditations, and nutritional and herbal support. When you nurture yourself daily, you increase your self-awareness throughout the day, notice your energy, treat your feelings and emotions with tenderness, and are mindful of your thoughts and mental patterns. Ultimately, Daily Self-Care, Special Healing Treats, and Easing the Lines of Life will allow you to touch and care for all aspects of yourself as your own flow of life force unites with the source of all life.

These rituals are not a fleeting fancy of exercises that you will use once and discard. They are designed to introduce you to your self, to help you experience the fullness of who you are. These are not throwaway moments. Allow yourself the gift of a moment of your full attention, the gift of your loving and tender touch, the gift of nurturing and allowing your inner radiance to come forward and face the world.

5. DAILY RITUALS

STAYING PRESENT TO EACH AND EVERY MOMENT OF OUR LIFE IS THE ULTIMATE ACT OF SELF-CARE. WITH THE WORLD CONSTANTLY DEMANDING OUR ATTENTION, WE NEED SIMPLE WAYS TO REPLENISH EACH ASPECT OF OURSELVES. OUTER BEAUTY AND INNER PEACE DEPEND ON THE SYNCHRONIZATION OF ALL LEVELS OF BEING.

Self-care, self-help, do-it-yourself—we are all familiar with these terms. At its most basic level, self-care means caring for the hygienic needs of the body. However, as we have already described in this book, the self may be far more than you ever dreamed. Self-care needs to encompass all the things you do for yourself, not just physical care of the body and its pains, traumas, knots, and strains. Your self encompasses your feelings and emotions, your mind and thoughts, your intuition and energy, and your spirit as well as your body. The body is the point of power, the point where all the levels converge.

This awareness brings the realization that self-care must touch and nurture all aspects of your self. Each ritual is designed to bring your awareness to the wholeness of who you are and bring forward your essential beauty every day. Some rituals take only a moment, others several minutes. Some can be done throughout the day, while others will be more effective if you create the quiet space for inner communion.

Each ritual will assist you in beginning or continuing:

- to support the flows of energy throughout your body;

- to be tender with your feelings as you move through your day;

- to be mindful of your thoughts and mental patterns;

- to connect with the source of all life and bring that life force to all you do.

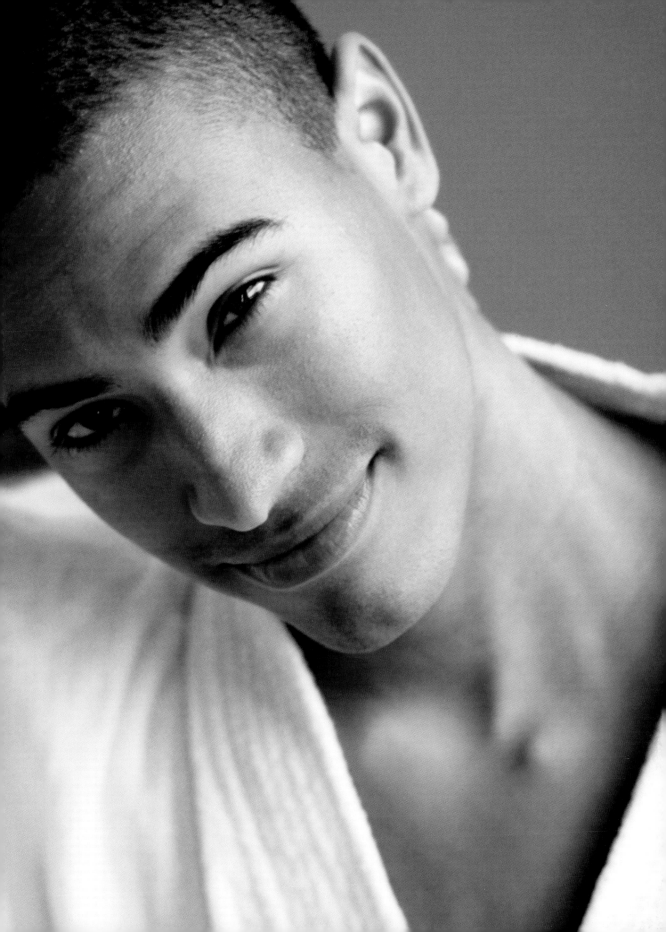

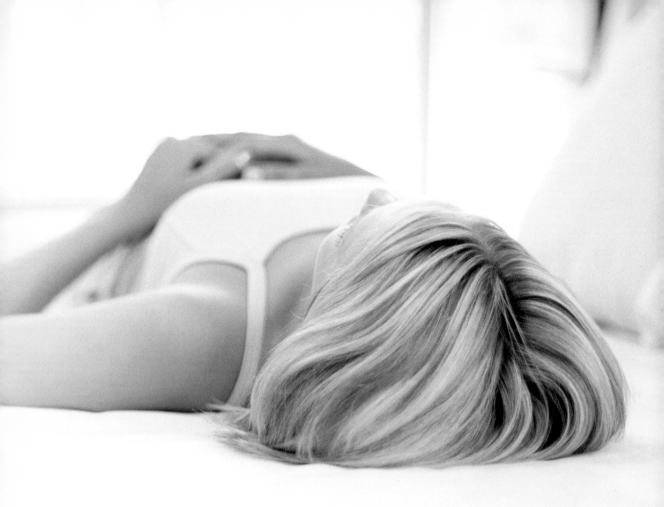

WAKE UP AND FACE THE DAY—
MORNING RITUALS

We stumble out of bed every morning, trailing our dreams, mobilizing our energy to

move into the day. Most of our early morning habits are so deeply entrenched that

we can almost do them with our eyes still closed. Today, you can begin a new routine.

By altering your morning habits and bringing more consciousness to the process of

waking up, you can present your best face to the day ahead.

Wake Up and Face the Day is a five-part routine that wakes up more than your

body. It also wakes up your vital energy, emotional balance, and mental clarity.

It attunes you to your highest self. Each part can be done independently, but the entire

routine takes less than 15 minutes and can be completed before your morning shower.

WAKE UP YOUR BODY

The first few moments of consciousness can set the tone for the rest of your day. In that delicious transition between sleep and waking—while you are still wrapped in the warmth and comfort of your pillows and covers—begin this stretch. Gentle stretching allows the energetic flows in the physical systems of the body to reestablish themselves. As you feed your cellular structures with loving attention, energy follows thought. When you get out of bed, you will feel more alive.

1. Breathe in deeply. Bring your attention to your body and roll over onto your back.

2. With slow, deliberate movements, rotate your hands and wrists several times in each direction. Feel the rotation all through your hands and forearms.

3. Stretch out to either side with arms and hands, opening first your chest and then your back widely. Allow yourself a luscious, enlivening stretch, arching your back, rolling your shoulders, and then relaxing completely.

4. Breathe in deeply the possibility of your day, and exhale all your concerns.

5. Now focus on your ankles and, with slow, deliberate movements, rotate your feet several times in each direction. Feel the rotation all through your feet and calves while your toes wiggle and stretch.

6. Stretch downward by pointing your toes. Stretch your legs from ankle to hips, tightening your buttocks and lifting the pelvis slightly. Hold for a moment, then relax completely.

7. Flex each foot, pressing down through your heels. Alternate feet, flexing first one, then the other. Feel the stretch in your hips as your leg muscles lengthen. Flex your feet together again and feel the lengthening of your spine. Relax completely.

8. Throw off the covers and bring your knees to your chest. Hug them with your arms, giving the spine a soft curve. Gently rock your hips from side to side. Relax completely in this position.

9. Roll onto your side and sit up slowly.

10. Roll your neck slowly—clockwise and counterclockwise—before standing up.

WAKE UP YOUR VITAL ENERGY—HOT LEMON JUMP START

This warm and enlivening drink is a great substitute for—or prelude to—morning coffee. It is also a wonderful pick-me-up for the afternoon. Lemon juice helps to complete the digestion of yesterday's meals while it refreshes and alkalinizes the digestive system. Organic honey adds essential minerals and enzymes. Grade B maple syrup is high in mineral content and is a soothing reminder of morning treats. Powdered cayenne pepper and fresh ginger are amazing healing herbs for the whole body. Cayenne is high in nutrition and therapeutically stimulating for the blood, lymph, digestive enzymes, and vital energy flows. Fresh ginger is a gentler stimulant for these systems and warms the body's chi.

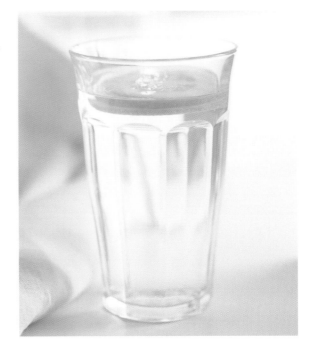

1. Into 1 cup (236 ml) of hot water, stir:
- the juice of $^1/_2$ an organic lemon, and
- 1–2 teaspoons of organic honey or grade B maple syrup.

2. Top with a light sprinkle of cayenne pepper or a bit of grated fresh ginger.

3. Sip and enjoy before you eat anything else.

While you wait for the water to boil for the hot lemon jump start, sit in a chair for a few moments and use the Rejuv Touch to wake up your mind with clarity and creativity.

In this touch routine, you will concentrate on the pituitary gland, the physical plant manager of your body. The pituitary manages the body's metabolic functions. It tells your body what to do, when to do it, and how to do it. The touch at the forehead accesses the pituitary directly and stimulates its functioning. It also stimulates the activity of your third eye, or sixth chakra— the energy center that controls clear vision, perception, and focus. The touch at the temple points accesses the pituitary along the winged expansion of the sphenoid bone. This touch adds an expanded peripheral dimension and clarity to your vision. Adding the vibration of the color yellow (using traditional color therapy) provides clarifying frequencies to brain functions and thinking processes.

Wake up your mind as you start your day with this ritual. You can also use this technique as a quick focusing tool to generate clarity about any personal or professional project.

1. Sit comfortably with your back straight. Place the index and middle fingertips of each hand on the pituitary point in your third eye area. Hold this position.

2. Repeat the Rejuv Breath (see Chapter 4), bringing in the color yellow. Choose any shade from soft butter to neon yellow or simply a clear light.

3. Inhale to a slow count of three, filling your entire body with your color for this morning.

4. Exhale to a slow count of three, radiating this color out into your auric field.

5. Inhale to a slow count of three, bathing your lungs.

6. Exhale to a slow count of three, radiating this color out into your auric field.

7. Inhale to a slow count of three, saturating your head.

8. Exhale to a slow count of three, radiating this color out into your auric field.

9. Without releasing your fingertips, lightly touch your thumbs to your temple points.

10. Repeat the three Rejuv color breaths as above.

11. Release your hands and sit quietly for a few moments.

12. If you have a special project today, bring it to mind and bathe it in this bright clarity. You will approach it with clear intention and creative energy.

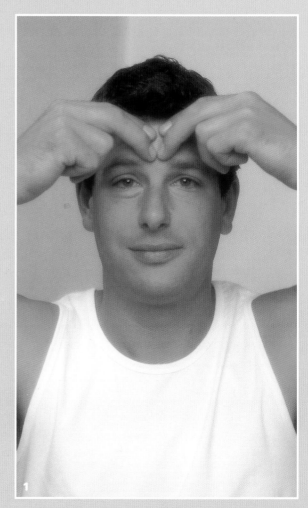

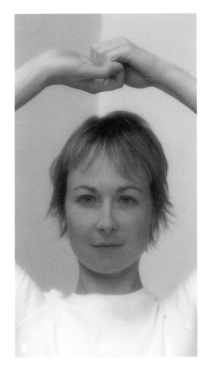

After relaxing and drinking your hot lemon jump start, bring your attention to your emotions. The Coupler Pull is a simple technique to bring your emotions, mind, and body into harmony. It can be used any time you feel out of balance or off center.

1. To begin, check the length of your hands and fingers by lining up the creases on your wrists and melting your hands together: heels, palms, fingers. If you are out of balance, one hand's fingertips will generally appear slightly longer than the other.

2. Bring both hands in front of you at chest level.

3. With one palm up and the other palm down, interlock your curled fingers like the coupler between the cars of a train.

4. Pull your hands apart with just enough tension for a firm hold. Maintain the pull as you continue.

5. Inhale, raising hands above your head, maintaining the pull. Hold for a count of seven.

6. Exhale, bringing your hands down, maintaining the pull. Release your fingers and switch hand position. Interlock curled fingers and repeat as above.

7. Inhale, raising your hands above your head and maintaining the pull. Hold for a count of seven.

8. Exhale, bringing your hands down, maintaining the pull. Release your fingers.

9. Check the length of your hands and fingers. Your hands and fingers should now be the same length.

WAKE UP TO YOURSELF—BIG SLURP

The Big Slurp brings awareness to the thought that we are all connected. Alignment, centeredness, balance, and connection are all qualities that help a day go well. This simple technique helps create a physical and energetic connection between our energy system or chakras and our glandular system. By bringing us to center, it helps balance the flow between the systems and connect our inner and outer spaces—the link between our body and the universe. When all aspects of the self are balanced and in tune, we have clear access to our highest potential in the moment and throughout the day to come.

1. Bring to your mind's eye the seven chakras located in your physical-energetic body, the eighth chakra located a foot (about 30 cm) above your head, and the infinite space above that.

2. With the fingers of the right hand on the front of your body, touch the area of each chakra in order: the first (or root) chakra on your pubic bone, the second chakra on your lower abdomen, the third chakra on your solar plexus, the fourth on your heart, the fifth on your throat, the sixth on the third eye in the center of your forehead, and the seventh on the crown of your head.

3. Lift your hand a foot (about 30 cm) above your head to connect your body to the eighth chakra (soul potential) and release the line above you to the universe. Draw the line again, this time holding your hand 2 inches (5 cm) from your body and extending it above to the eighth chakra and beyond. Allow the energy of this line to align all your systems—physical, energetic, emotional, mental, and spiritual.

4. Imagine you are finishing a thick, rich ice cream soda; you need a big slurp to get the last bit of ice cream up through the straw. Feel the sensation.

5. Now, imagine a straw at your root chakra. Duplicate the sensation, as you slurp the goodness of who you are up through each chakra, from root to crown and out into the universe.

6. Breathe into this alignment, allowing your body to shift slightly, sitting tall at the center of all that you are.

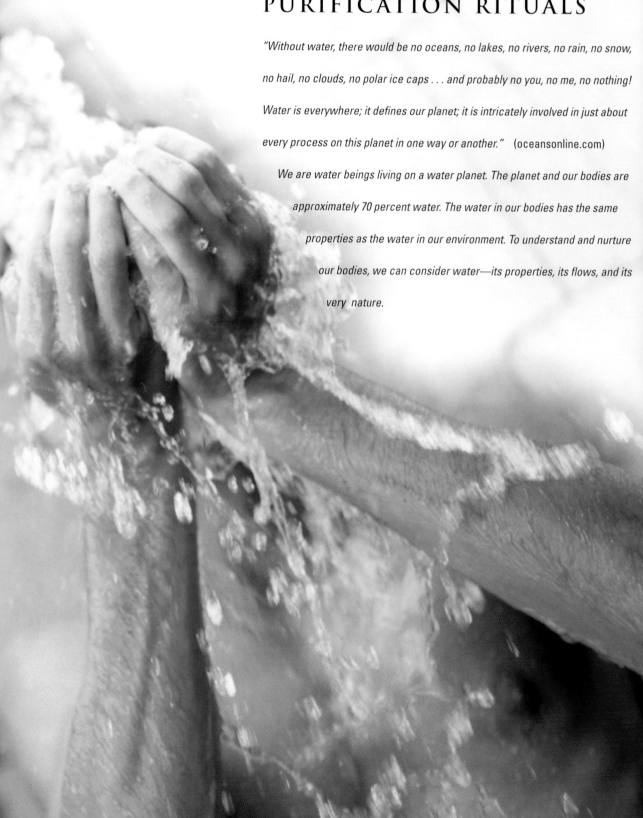

WATER RITES—
PURIFICATION RITUALS

"Without water, there would be no oceans, no lakes, no rivers, no rain, no snow, no hail, no clouds, no polar ice caps . . . and probably no you, no me, no nothing! Water is everywhere; it defines our planet; it is intricately involved in just about every process on this planet in one way or another."   (oceansonline.com)

We are water beings living on a water planet. The planet and our bodies are approximately 70 percent water. The water in our bodies has the same properties as the water in our environment. To understand and nurture our bodies, we can consider water—its properties, its flows, and its very nature.

THE ESSENTIAL POWER OF WATER

Water is a human necessity. It can be a sustaining substance, cradling an infant in the womb, or a powerful force, eroding rocks one drop at a time and aiding in the creation of the Grand Canyon. Whether water sustains or erodes, solvency is the key to its strength and our need for plenty of it.

Water is considered a universal solvent because almost any substance can be dissolved into it. The water, full of elemental substances, travels and moves those substances from point to point. On Earth this transport happens through rain, streams, rivers, and oceans. In our bodies, the flow of water in blood and lymph brings nourishment to every cell and transports toxins to be eliminated.

This happens on the physical level. However, it is not just a poetic notion that water is a potent and deeply moving presence in our lives. Beyond its physical effects, water also represents the flows of our higher vibratory levels, the flows of our meridian systems, the flows of our mercurial emotions, and even the flows of our unending streams of thought.

Given the essential nature of water, both within and without us, Water Rites elevate these rituals to the spaciousness and sacred time they deserve. How we interact with the water we drink, the water we bathe in, even the water in which we wash our dishes will ultimately change and renew our connection to the very flows of the life force that animate us.

SHOWER OF LIGHT AND COLOR

You do not need special equipment, fancy lighting, or a new bathroom—just add your imagination to your daily shower to create a watery flow of light and color. By using the image of water's solvent properties, you dissolve and carry away all that is no longer needed on any level of your being. Feel the inner experience of release and cleansing. You can also do this as an inner practice during meditation or to rebalance yourself at any point during your day. Be creative—add stretching, movement, and breath to assist the release and absorption of the light and color. This ritual provides a great focus during a morning run or exercise routine.

1. Focus on the intersection of the midline and coronal planes (see Chapter 3).

2. Let your breath bring awareness to all the levels of your being: from your core, through your body to your skin and beyond to encompass your auric field.

3. Imagine a shower nozzle several feet above your head, ready to shower you with light and color. Turn on this cosmic shower, and let this moment's perfect intensity of light and color stream through you. Be aware of the color or colors as they flow through your head to your feet and beyond you into Earth.

4. Allow the shower of light and color to wash away all static, stress, and tension.

5. If you are in the shower, use the water to carry the light and color around your body and imagine it flowing through you.

6. Notice any places where the light or color seems to get stuck, then bring more flow of both into the area. When you feel the release is complete, let yourself absorb the light and color. Delight in the beauty and the flow available to you. You may feel yourself tingle with life force as you fully absorb it.

7. When you feel the stream of light and color flowing unimpeded, turn off the cosmic shower, take a deep breath, and give yourself a full-body stretch.

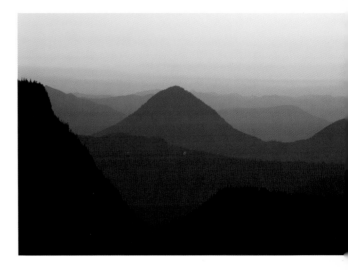

Since it was so hard to come by in ancient times, water was more treasured then than it is today. An honored guest would be greeted with a washing and anointing of the feet. Today we will greet our own feet with a ritual that is rooted in this cleansing and blessing ceremony.

Soaking your feet for 20 minutes will hydrate and refresh you. The solvency properties of water will absorb the tensions and chaotic nerve signals from feet that have supported your weight throughout the day. The powerful healing influence of water can be increased by adding herbs or essential oils to the soak.

Completing the ritual with a six-minute foot rub not only eases tired feet but restores energy to your whole body through the ancient art of foot reflexology. By simply

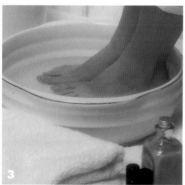

rubbing your feet, you stimulate nerve endings on the foot, sending impulses along the length of the nerve fiber throughout the body. You do not have to be a skilled foot reflexology practitioner to receive the benefits of a simple foot rub. You do not even need to know which areas of the foot correspond to specific organ systems; just trust your intuition.

EQUIPMENT/ MATERIALS

• A large basin with enough hot water to cover both feet above the ankles.

• A pitcher of extra hot water.

• Two fluffy towels.

• Your choice of essential oils. Try one of the following: sage for circulation, rosemary for clarity, lemon for cooling, or lavender for relaxing.

• Your choice of foot balm: an organic oil, cream, or lotion.

Optional: See "baths" and use the same ingredients for a foot soak.

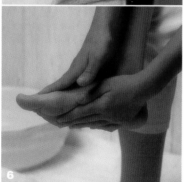

1. Begin by scheduling your time (at least 30 minutes) and preparing your space (chair/bowl) to soak and greet your feet.

2. Add 4–8 drops of essential oil to the water, then seat yourself comfortably.

3. Slip your feet into the fragrant, steaming water. Lean back and allow the footbath to begin activating all of your reflexology points.

4. Soak until the water starts cooling, 20–30 minutes. If you have more time, add more hot water.

5. Dry your feet and remove the basin before applying foot balm.

6. Gently massage the foot balm into all areas of each foot. Deeply and slowly massage each foot. Do not forget your toes and heels.

7. If an area is sore, hold the point with full presence (see Chapter 4) until you feel a shift in the point, then release and continue massaging.

8. If you bring your full presence and care to your feet, even 2–3 minutes on each foot can be of great benefit to your entire system.

9. When you have completed both feet, curl and stretch the toes and rotate your feet at the ankles. Relax and enjoy the feeling before continuing your activities.

ELIXIR OF LIFE

When we apply an elementary understanding of quantum physics to water molecules, we realize that there is memory in its subatomic structures. Whether it is crashing on a deserted beach, frozen in a snowflake, or steaming from a hot tub—water remembers.

Whenever we take in water—in any form—we can use its ability to retain information. You can imprint the water to hold healing and revitalizing energy. You can use the following procedure to energize any water and anything that has water in it—which includes almost everything you eat and drink. Magnetizing water with intention on a daily basis can have far-reaching and profound possibilities to refresh and renew you at the cellular level.

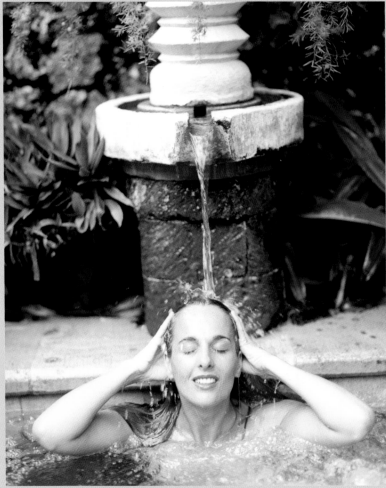

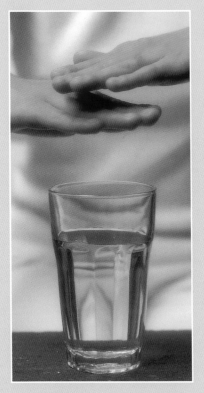

1. Pour a glass of water (begin with pure water before expanding to other drinks and foods). Take a sip and notice how the water tastes and feels before you begin.

2. Place your right palm chakra over the glass.

3. Align your left palm chakra over the right.

4. Hold the position, chakra over chakra, energy center over energy center, always right first, then left.

5. Focus your intention and energy through your palm chakras to energize and magnetize the water with healing frequencies.

6. See, feel, or imagine pure positive energy flowing into the water. You can use a ray of light, a color, a warm glow, or simply a good feeling that arises naturally.

7. Hold this position for 30–60 seconds or as long as you feel guided to effect a change.

8. Relax your hands, then lift the glass and drink the water.

9. Notice any changes, tastes, or sensations as you drink.

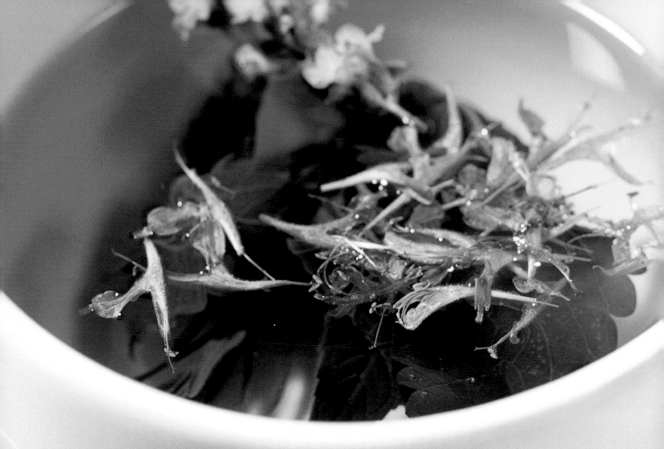

NON-COFFEE BREAKS—
RECHARGING RITUALS

We usually think of a coffee break as a time to recharge our batteries with a quick fix.

This time often occurs sometime between breakfast and lunch and again when we are

slumping in the middle of the afternoon. The following recharging rituals will provide

alternatives to the caffeine and sugar high that leaves our inner systems in worse condition

than before the break. These rituals are quick and provide a real kick by giving the body the

raw materials to produce the energy you need.

The first indication that your body needs some help is a general craving. Your first

response should be to drink water. Remember, it is the elixir of life after a few seconds under

your loving attention. Then add another of the following suggestions. Try them all and use

your favorites as daily support for your inner and outer beauty.

Both drinks can be used at any time, but their specific nutrients are designed to bring the body to balance in different ways.

Cayenne punch

Cayenne pepper is a valuable nutritive aid to increasing wellness in the body and mind; it is also a convenient and gentle stimulant to your circulation and energy flows. Adding as little as a sprinkle of raw, powdered cayenne pepper to a tasty liquid on a daily basis aids digestion, circulation, and nerve integrity. Cayenne provides a surge of clarity and helps sustain your concentration and focus. Cayenne pepper is packed with vitamins and minerals and is a superb alternative to the debilitating spike and crash of the caffeine in coffee.

1. Start slowly (just a sprinkle) if you are not used to hot spices. Work up to $1/4$ to $1/2$ teaspoon of powdered cayenne in juice.

2. When combined with grape juice, cayenne pepper builds the blood and serves as an herbal stimulant, giving your system the "juice" it needs to stay awake and focused. (This is an excellent dietary aid for those who are sometimes anemic.)

3. When combined with tomato juice, it adds a blast of clarity that lasts. OPTION: Sprinkle it on everything! It may be fierce in your mouth at first, but as an herbal demulcent, cayenne will soothe all your internal tissues as it stimulates organ function.

Green drink

This simple drink is a powerhouse of bioavailable nutrition. It contains everything your body needs to kickstart your day or to revive your system in the afternoon. The deep green color is from chlorophyll-rich parsley filled with essential vitamins and minerals. Although any combination of nuts and seeds you use will provide a power pack of slightly different nutrition, always use protein-rich almonds as the base. While the nuts and seeds soak overnight, their nutritional potential explodes as germination begins. This allows the load of proteins, vitamins, minerals, and essential fatty acids to be readily assimilated. The addition of pineapple juice provides bromelain, an enzyme that assists the digestion of all the nutrients in the drink. This green shake is rich and delicious—do not let the color put you off.

1. Soak eight almonds and your choice of nuts and seeds ($1/2$ to 1 teaspoon of each: sunflower, sesame, flax, pumpkin, chia) in water overnight. Be sure the container leaves room for them to swell.

2. In the morning, blend with $1/2$ cup (125 ml) pineapple juice (unsweetened, NOT from concentrate).

3. Add fresh parsley (organic whenever possible) until the blend turns green (about $1/3$ of a regular-sized bunch).

4. Add more pineapple juice, if necessary, to bring the mixture to your preferred consistency.

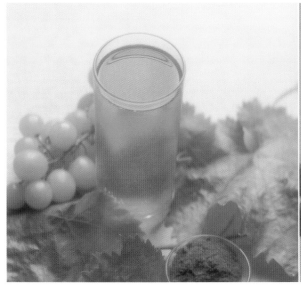

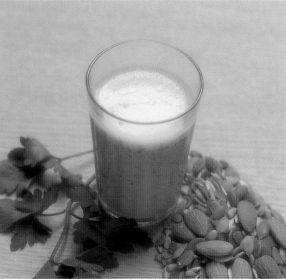

MAGIC BUTTONS

We all know about those hidden emotional triggers that appear when someone pushes our buttons. The body also has a few buttons that can trigger positive flows to the entire system, bringing balance to the mind and body. We have already explored the relief available through foot reflexology, the following rituals access other powerful points.

Adrenal fatigue is a common condition today. The simple pattern of breathe and hold allows the adrenals to discharge some of the subliminal exhaustion and re-boot themselves. These hand reflexology points are easy to use, at any time of stress or fatigue. Massaging several times a day will begin to diminish the back load of adrenal fatigue and the adrenal glands can begin to replenish. The adrenal glands mobilize us on physiological, energetic, and emotional levels to protect and defend ourselves inwardly and outwardly—they are our fight-or-flight directors. Their optimal function supports health body-wide.

ADRENAL INFUSION

1. Use the thumb of one hand to stimulate the adrenal gland in the center of the palm chakra of the other hand.

2. Gently massage this area, the adrenal contact point.

3. Inhale and hold the point as you hold your breath (breathe and hold).

4. Release and exhale. Repeat three times.

5. Switch to the opposite thumb and hand and also reposition.

6. Massage the area of the adrenal contact on the second hand.

7. Breathe and hold three times.

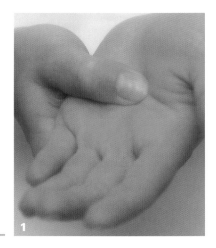

HEAD-TAPPING

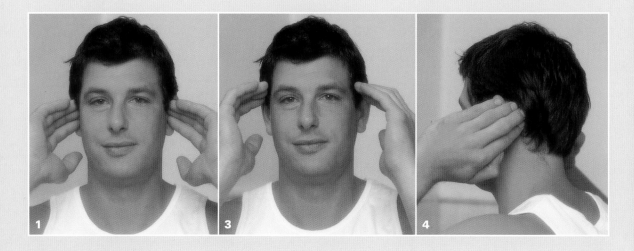

HEAD-TAPPING

Tapping necessitates a loose wrist that allows the soft but quick contact of bone-to-bone percussion. This gentle stimulation activates nerve centers, meridians, and the brain.

1. Begin with all four fingertips of each hand placed in front of your ears, middle fingers at the triangle ear points.

2. Begin tapping softly and quickly.

3. Tap upward into the temple area until the index finger taps there.

4. Continue tapping above and around the top of the ear, allowing your tapping fingertips to move downward onto the mastoid bone behind the ear.

5. Tap on this bone gently for a few seconds, longer than in the other areas. Your cupped hands will feel like seashells around your ears as you tap.

6. Continue tapping along the base of the skull (the occipital ridge) toward the midline.

7. Tap at the midline for a few extra moments, then return along the base of the skull until your index fingers are at the parotid points. Stop tapping.

8. Slide your hands down slightly and replace the index finger position with your middle fingertips. Hold the parotid points in stillness.

9. Close your eyes and take several deep breaths as you hold these points.

10. Gently lift your middle fingers and touch the temple points. Hold.

11. Gently lift your middle fingers and touch the pituitary point. Hold.

12. Gently lift your middle fingers and touch the crown of your head. Hold.

13. With your last inhalation, lift your hands off the crown with a gentle upward stretch.

14. With your last exhalation, sweep your hands in an arc through your auric field and rest them at your sides.

15. Become aware of the vital energy coursing through your mind and body.

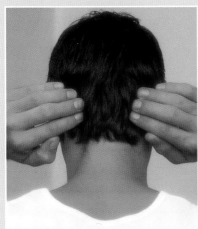
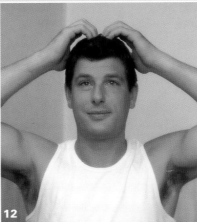
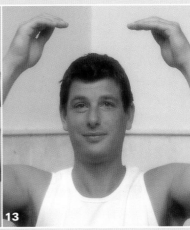

RELAX AND RELEASE THE DAY— EVENING RITUALS

Letting go of the day is an essential step in allowing sleep to fully nourish us. It is also critical to prepare for the new day and its fresh influx of sights, sounds, and situations. Our nightly routines can be as habitual as our morning routines. The following evening rituals can be added to the simple relaxation aids that we already know—the cup of chamomile blossom tea, the warm fragrant bath, or a long, hot shower. Create the time and space to wind down from the day's activities using the five-part routine to relax and release the day. Each part can be used independently. Together, though, they can become a new routine that prepares you for deep rest and renewal in as little as 15 minutes.

The Deep Soothe brings you home to your self. Because your palms are outlining your body's hills and hollows with acute sensory awareness, you are defining your physical container—the grounding point that integrates all your levels of being. This simple wipe off frees the parasympathetic nervous system from the excessive signaling load from the day. Once released of this static charge, the body is more easily nourished by food and drink as well as by the flows of cosmic energy. You can spend as little as two minutes or a long, luscious ten minutes on yourself or with another. The Deep Soothe can be done dressed or undressed, either sitting or standing. Each wipe off is done three times moving from the core to the periphery and ending with a flick of the wrist into the energy field. Create your magnetic mitts as below.

Front

1. Begin with both hands at your heart.

2. Wipe up the midline, following the contours of the chest, neck, and face, wiping off through the hair to the crown and into the energy field. Flick.

3. Opposite hands do each arm. Begin at the heart and wipe up to the shoulder, down the arm to the hand and wipe off at the fingers. Flick.

4. Wipe off from midline toward the coronal plane from the forehead to pelvis. Flick.

5. Begin with both hands on the abdomen and wipe down the legs to the feet and wipe off at the toes. Flick.

Back

6. Begin with both hands on lower back, following the contours of the buttocks, thighs, calves. Wipe down to your heel. Flick.

7. Wipe off from midline toward the coronal plane from the buttocks to the mid-back. Flick.

8. Begin with both hands at the back of the neck (as low as is comfortable), wipe up the midline of the back, neck, head. Wipe off through the hair to the crown and into the energy field. Flick.

To End

9. Rest in stillness and be aware of your body.

MAGNETIC MITTS TO DE-STRESS THE BODY

Your palms are energy centers that radiate an electro-magnetic field. You can increase this radiation and allow your hands to become magnetic healing mitts.

1. Inhale deeply and gently, using the Rejuv Breath (see Chapter 4).

2. Exhale, sending the breath down your arms, into your hands, and out through your palms.

3. Repeat the breathing pattern until you feel/sense/imagine that your palms are ready.

4. Slowly wipe your mitts over your entire body.

5. Imagine you are magnetically collecting excess static charge of negative energy from each area.

6. Wipe with slow, deliberate, conscious movements.

7. Disperse the energy off each mitt with a flick of the wrist.

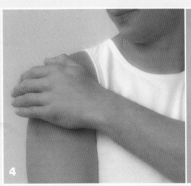
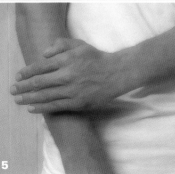
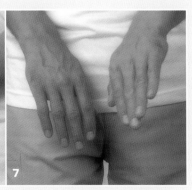

Our vital energy system is as complex as our physical system; its major "organs" are the chakras. We need to nourish the chakra system with as much care and attention as we give to our physical body. The food, water, and air for our energetic system is awareness, consciousness, prana, and breath. The elimination and release of what is no longer serving us is equally important to both systems. Daily attention to our energetic needs supports our physical, emotional, and spiritual health.

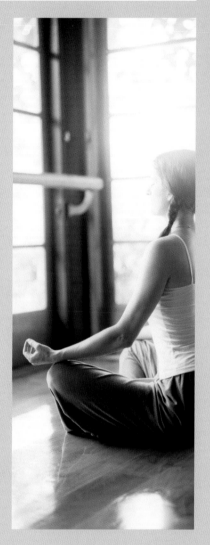

1. Breathe gently and easily in your own rhythm, bringing your awareness to the line and flow of your chakra system.

2. Bring your attention to your first chakra—the root—and see/feel/imagine yourself within this chakra.

3. Create a chute of light from the bottom of the chakra deep into Earth.

4. Look around, sensing what you need to release, and let go of everything and anything within this chakra that limits your balance, wholeness, and connection to the divine.

5. Give yourself permission to begin the process of release; let deep cleanse begin, using any of the chakra cleaning techniques. Feel the draining happening.

6. When all is clean and clear, move up to the next chakra.

7. Create a chute of light in this chakra and connect it to the one below, then repeat the deep cleanse procedure.

8. Continue with each chakra until the eighth chakra, the one above the crown chakra.

9. Let all your chakras simultaneously open wide, allowing a fresh prana-filled breeze to enliven, balance, and refresh the entire system.

10. Let the breeze blow through your chakras for as long as it feels appropriate.

11. Allow these windows to close gently.

12. Breathe through the fullness of your entire chakra system with a sense of wholeness and inner connection.

CHAKRA CLEANING TECHNIQUES

This is where cleaning takes no time at all—and it can be fun! Keep it light and playful. Be creative; use some of these ideas or make up your own.

1. Bring in anything or anyone to help you do a bang-up cleaning job.

2. Vacuum the space with a high volume vacuum cleaner.

3. Bring in your favorite superhero or comic book character to clean the closets.

4. Invite rainbow-colored dragons, angels, or fairies to burn off the impurities, dump them down a "chute of light" and leave iridescent sparkles everywhere.

5. Gather all the old and excessive stuff in nets of starlight and whisk it all down the chute.

RELAX YOUR MIND—A TOUCH OF CALM

A Touch of Calm is restorative to both mind and body. This touch sequence helps still the rapid-fire functions of the brain. Our thoughts weave complex tapestries of energy in and around us. Some of these threads are necessary and useful for moving us through the day. The threads of our incomplete thoughts leave us exhausted and push the brain to process them throughout the night. Rest and sleep are more accessible when the threads of our thoughts are untangled.

1. Sit comfortably with your back straight.

2. Place the index and middle fingertips of each hand on the temple points. Hold.

3. Repeat the Rejuv Breath three times to bring in a color: lavender, indigo, or rose. Choose any shade you may be drawn to this evening.

4. Inhale to a slow count of three, saturating your head with color.

5. Exhale to a slow count of three, radiating this color out into your auric field.

6. Inhale to a slow count of three, bathing your throat area (fifth chakra).

7. Exhale to a slow count of three, radiating this color out into your auric field.

8. Inhale to a slow count of three, filling your entire body.

9. Exhale to a slow count of three, radiating this color out into your auric field.

10. Release the temples and place the middle fingertips of each hand onto the parotid points. Hold.

11. Repeat the three Rejuv Color Breaths as above.

12. Release the parotid points and place your hands onto your heart center, first right palm, then left palm. Hold.

13. Repeat the three Rejuv Color Breaths as above.

14. Release your hands and breathe quietly for a few moments.

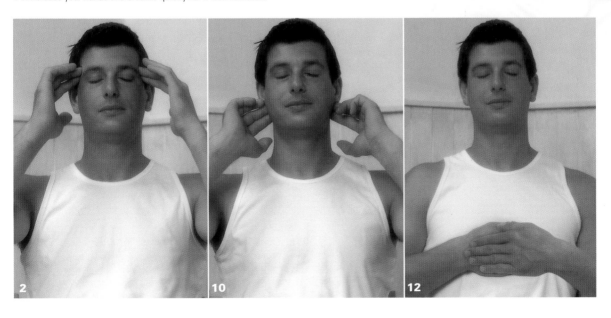

After calming your conscious thoughts, spend some time releasing your emotional connections to the day. Neutrality does not mean that we do not care; it means that we are not easily swayed by our emotional reactions. Moving through the day with neutrality allows us to receive the gifts and enjoy the challenges presented to us. This meditation gives us the opportunity to look over the day as a neutral observer, taking in the gifts more fully and releasing any residual discomfort.

1. Begin with a few deep breaths into the bowl of your pelvis, centering into the core of your self.

2. Let your breath settle into an easy rhythm.

3. Allow the feelings and situations from the day flow into your mind.

4. If an image is positive, place your hands, first the right, then the left, over your heart center.

5. Let yourself absorb the positive image to increase your feelings of satisfaction or delight. Let your heart be fed by this image as you "eat" the positive energy flow and enjoy it.

6. When you have fully harvested the goodness of that moment, release your hands and let another image surface.

7. If an image is negative, cup your fingertips into a C and tap gently around the temple points, from the top to the bottom in a C curve, four to five times.

8. When you feel the tension soften, lower your hands and breathe deeply, allowing the emotional crystallizations loosened by the tapping to dissolve as you breathe.

9. Continue reviewing the day, absorbing and releasing, until the day's images and memories slow down within you.

10. Feel the balance point of neutrality and poise start to stabilize and increase. Rest in this place.

11. Open your eyes and enjoy the emotional relaxation, having truly completed your day.

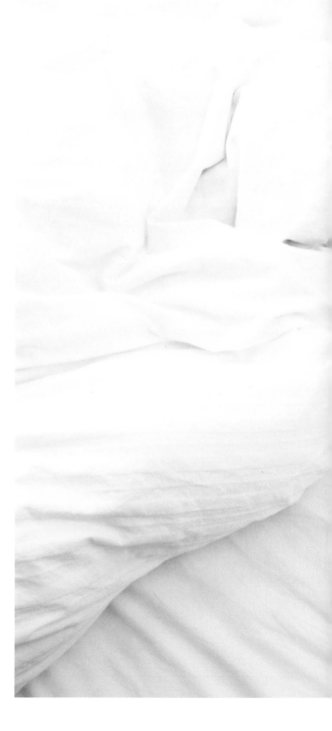

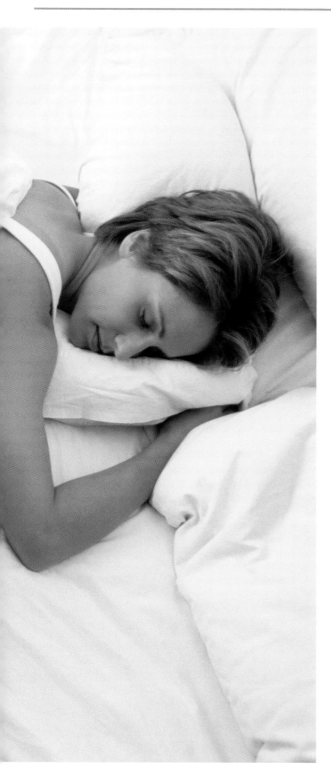

How do you prepare for sleep? A hot toddy, a few pages from a book, another movie on cable? Notice how your nightly routine affects your sleep. If you have used the first four rituals to release the day, you may not need this last nightcap. If you use only this meditation, take the time to make it your own, encompassing all the other components. Use it to spark your imagination and clear the energies of the day in more holistic ways.

Once you have relaxed and released the day using the first four rituals, take time to create a cocoon of warmth and safety for sleep. Preparing yourself and your space in this way will allow your body to rest more deeply, having been replenished and refreshed by the divine life force.

1. Tuck yourself into your bed. However, before you curl into your favorite position, lie flat on your back.

2. Focus on your breath and notice any places of tension or discomfort in your body.

3. While inhaling, tighten the area and release it as you exhale.

4. Track your entire body, tightening and releasing until you feel body-wide relaxation.

5. Focus on your breath and notice your energy centers, the chakras.

6. Use your breath to harmonize each chakra with a color. You can use the colors that are associated with each chakra or create your own unique palette (first—red, second—orange, third—yellow, fourth—green, fifth—blue, sixth—indigo, seventh—purple, eighth—clear).

7. Focus on your breath and notice your mind and emotions.

8. Use acceptance and forgiveness as you breathe to bring each thought and emotion into a space of peace. Allow the day to be exactly what it was and let it go.

9. Breathe gently, becoming aware of all the dimensions of your self.

10. See, feel, or imagine a color, shape, or sound that brings a sense of security and comfort to you tonight.

11. Be creative—paint the entire room in a rainbow of colors, put a cube or a pyramid of light around the bed, imagine angels or guardians of sleep at the four corners, hear a wind chime or the ocean in the distance. Lay a soft, warm blanket of light over your body, and wrap yourself in it.

12. Hold the image until it feels stable and real. Rest in it.

13. Settle into your favorite sleeping position.

6. SPECIAL HEALING TREATS

SPECIAL HEALING TREATS IS THE PERFECT NAME FOR ALL THE RITUALS CONTAINED WITHIN THIS CHAPTER. SPECIAL BECAUSE THEY ARE OFTEN-FORGOTTEN LUXURIES THAT WE USUALLY DOLE OUT SPARINGLY. HEALING BECAUSE THEY ARE EFFECTIVE IN SUPPORTING WELLNESS IN BODY, MIND, AND SPIRIT. TREATS BECAUSE THEY ARE GIFTS WE CAN GIVE OURSELVES REGULARLY WITH DELIGHT AND EASE.

We begin with the bath, a luxurious necessity that can simulate a vacation in a mere 20 minutes. Adding a special ingredient to the bath can transform it into a healing moment, thus increasing the effective functioning of our physical and energetic structures. Any downtime we spend in a hot bath will be relaxing. However, by spending at least 20 minutes, we reap the most benefits from the energetic exchange of natural ingredients through our electromagnetic field. Twenty minutes is the magic time it takes for this exchange to occur.

Next, we will explore nutritional masks. Our faces can never be hidden from the world; every day they are seen by all. We want our faces to represent us in the very best way. The 20-minute magic of an organic facial treat can add an extra glow to every complexion. A variety of ingredients can aid the healing of dryness or patchy skin, improve overall circulation, exfoliate, and stimulate new cell regeneration.

We will conclude with multilevel support for those special occasions when we need a little extra TLC (tender loving care). Giving even a little attention to each level of our being can bring us into greater wholeness. A balanced protocol of simple techniques provides us with the tools to bring out our inner radiance and confidently face the future.

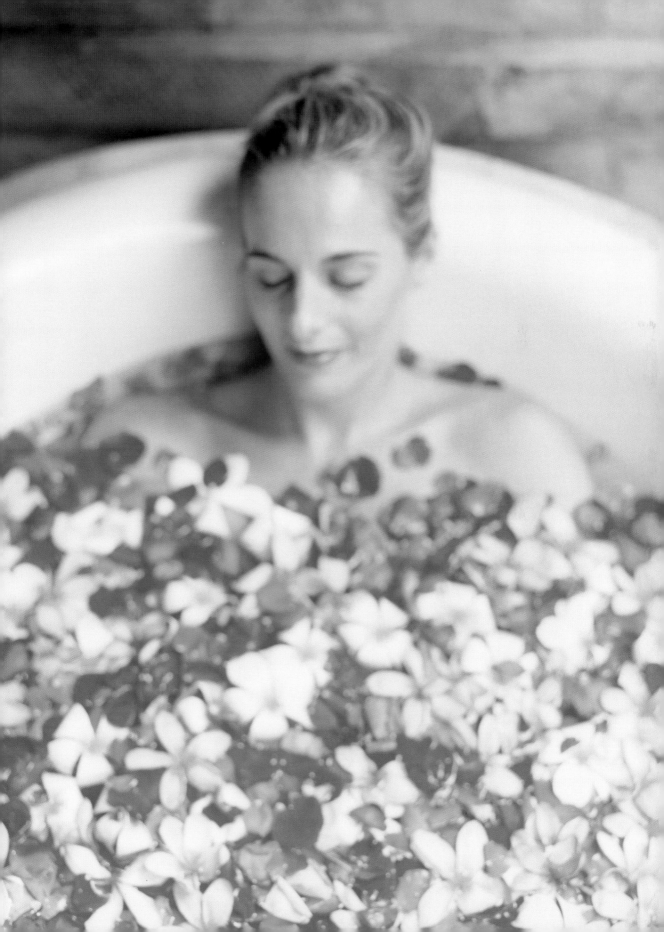

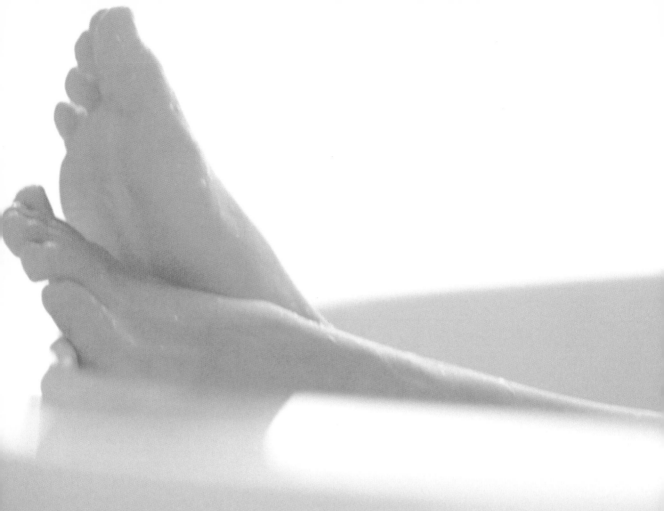

WATER WITHIN,
WATER WITHOUT

An emotion is said to be energy in motion. The chemical and electrical

components of our emotions travel throughout our bodies on the liquid

surface of hormones and nerves. This highly charged liquid energy also

flows though our auric envelope and affects our multilevel responses—

our words, our behaviors, our expressions, and even our intercellular

communication. Emotions are the watery element of our human nature.

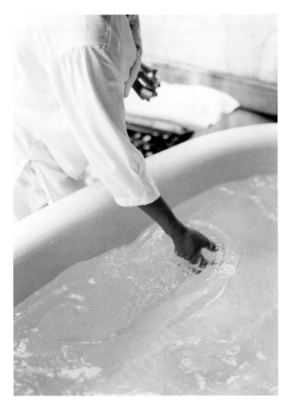

Although joy, peace, and harmony support internal balance, we are much more aware of the immediate response of human physiology to stress, fear, and anxiety. We can use the solvent nature of water to dilute and dissolve these tensions on every level. While soaking in a bath, you will experience your entire nervous system relaxing. Your adrenal glands, tiny glandular powerhouses that prepare you for "fight-or-flight," are definitely overworked by the intensity of modern daily life. The touch of warmth and water in the bath helps the body release its frenzy of activity and settle into deep inner communication and relaxation.

When approached mindfully, baths become a gentle and effective means to support all the aspects of our watery nature. The benefits of a prepared bath are many. Baths harmonize our inner and outer waters. They dissolve stress and tension, both emotional and physical, that may have accumulated during the day. A hot bath opens pores and promotes healthy sweating that draws environmental and metabolic toxins out of the body. Healing substances added to the water are absorbed through the open pores. Baths cleanse and stabilize the auric field. Immerse yourself as fully as possible in a bath of warm-to-hot water for 20 minutes or a luxurious hour. Sit back and relax; let the water do the work.

PSYCHIC STRESS RELEASE

Every day, we are bombarded by life's normal events. We have days that are slow and easy, others that are long and hard. Either way, we are subjected to a myriad of energetic frequencies that interact with our own. Psychic stress may feel as though we are carrying an unusually heavy load, feeling burdened and we may not know why. Psychic stress can be self-generated stress created by our thoughts, self-judgments, or lingering emotions, such as shame, anger, fear, or resentment. Although psychic stress can be absorbed in many ways from a situation, an environment, or an interaction, it can also be the simple residue of normal daily life.

There are many ways to clear your mind and release your emotions. To cleanse your energetic frequencies, the first choice is the Psychic Stress Release Bath. Just 1 cup (250 ml) of organic apple cider vinegar added to bathwater can help balance pH and rebuild your electromagnetic field. While soaking, you will feel the psychic load dissolve from your body, mind, and emotions. It cleans and refreshes the dumping ground of the auric field while detoxing negative energy from body. Use it to clear yourself any time, particularly in the early evening, to let go of the day and prepare for the evening's activities.

BATHTUB PREPARATION

1. Prepare a warm-to-hot bath.

2. Add 1 cup (250 ml) of organic apple cider vinegar.

3. Soak for 20 minutes, or for as long as you like.

4. Add more hot water and stay longer.

5. Showering after the bath is not necessary as the apple cider vinegar will restore the acid mantle of the skin.

MUSCLE TENSION-BUSTER

Ginger is packed with potent herbal healing and can be used internally or externally. This is the number one bath for overexertion of any kind. A 20-minute soak in a ginger bath is the antidote to almost any physical malaise. Take a muscle tension buster bath any time your muscles have stretched beyond their normal capacity, when you are bruised and exhausted, or when you have symptoms of a cold or flu.

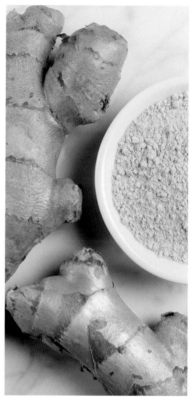

The heat of the ginger will promote sweating, allowing the pores to siphon off residual lactic acid from sore muscles. This heat helps stimulate circulation and relieve muscle pain, spasms, and cramps as toxins are released from the body. Drinking water during the soak is essential to promote sweating and to replace the water loss. You can use this bath to mitigate cold symptoms or a lukewarm bath to reduce fevers. A ginger bath can also relieve mosquito bites and other bug bites as well as heal welts. Taking this bath just before bedtime is best.

1. Prepare a very hot bath along with a glass of water to drink—you may wish to drink up to a quart (1 l) at room temperature.

2. Add 2 ounces (30 g) of powdered ginger to the tub if this is your first bath (for subsequent baths you can build up to 8 ounces [120 g] of ginger as the body becomes accustomed to its heat).

3. You may wish to sit on a washcloth because sitting on tiny bits of powered ginger can get rather intense.

4. Soak in the tub for at least 20 minutes or for as long as you like.

5. Add more hot water and stay longer.

6. Stand up slowly and wrap yourself in a big towel without rinsing first to allow the ginger to continue drawing out the toxins.

7. Put a robe on top of the towel and crawl into bed to continue sweating for at least another 20 minutes or until you start to cool down.

8. Dry off with a fresh towel (you may rinse yourself first if you prefer).

9. Prepare for bed and for a good night's sleep.

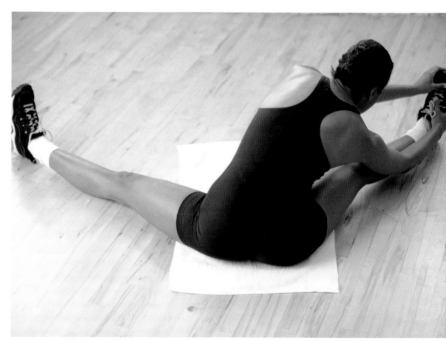

LUSCIOUS LEMON

We do not usually pay much attention to lemon's uplifting aroma when we squeeze its juice onto an entrée or drink a glass of lemonade. However, a simple strong whiff of lemon can elevate our mood, spinning our emotions gently in an upward spiral and holding them there. The essence of lemon in a bath does all that and more. Lusciously surrounding our entire body in the clean, crisp scent of lemon not only elevates our mood but also softens and soothes our skin.

A lemon bath cleanses the lymphatic system as it opens the pores and promotes perspiration. Lemon is also a strong antiseptic and a soothing, healing treatment for scaly, chapped, or scratched skin. As a daily aid for chapped hands, ragged cuticles, and rough elbows, keep a cut lemon by the kitchen sink and rub it into your hands and elbows after they have been immersed in water.

1. Prepare a hot bath.

2. Squeeze the juice from six fresh, organic lemons; discard the seeds.

3. Add the fresh juice and rinds of the lemons to the bath water.

4. Soak for at least 20 minutes or for as long as you like.

5. Add more hot water and stay longer.

6. Rinse off if you feel the need, but remember that the citric acid in the lemon helps restore the acid mantle of the skin. Be sure to discard the lemon rinds.

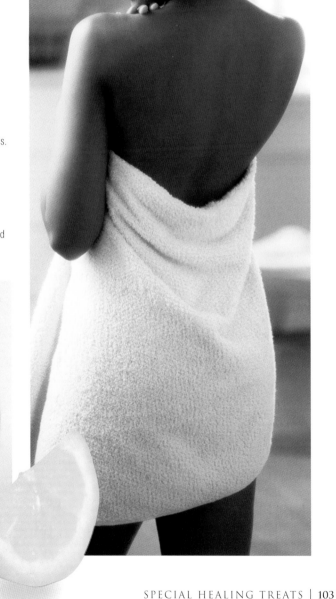

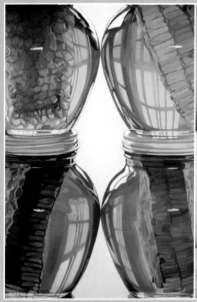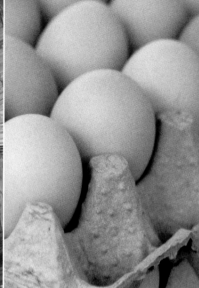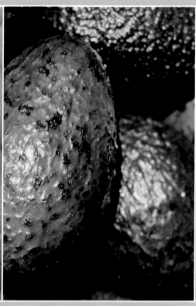

Natural Creations From the Kitchen

The four facial masks in this section are the result of years of experimentation on faces, backs, and necks by fine kitchen herbalists and natural healers. Use organic ingredients whenever possible to enhance the healing properties of each preparation. The choice of ingredients follows a simple rule—if you would not want to eat it, do not put it onto your face. The better the raw materials you use, the more effective the results.

Every cell in the body has a life cycle, and our skin cells are recreated every 14–21 days. Each mask is a "skin snack" designed to address different factors promoting cellular regeneration. As a general rule, leave these natural snacks on the face for 20 minutes. This amount of time will provide the necessary physical contact as well as the energetic exchange that will be most beneficial to your complexion.

You can use a wide variety of fruits and vegetables, nuts, seeds, and grains to make fabulous, natural facial masks. For the Deep Nourishment Mask, we have selected avocado. Grown in tropical climates, this lush fruit is filled with life force from the Sun, the sea, and salt-laden breezes. It conjures up the image of a healthy life attuned to Earth's cycles and the ripening of life-giving foods. Avocados contain a rich and varied cornucopia of nutrition and rejuvenating substances.

A honey of a rejuvenation facial cycle will create a three-week miracle for your face as it softens the effects of aging by improving the tone and texture of the skin. You will use one mask each day, rotating them in sequence for 21 days: Honey & Nutmeg, Cream & Honey, and Egg & Honey. These masks contain only four simple foods found in most kitchens. Elevate them to rich treasures by buying organic honey (unfiltered, unheated), organic eggs and cream, and fresh, whole nutmegs to truly feed your hungry skin. You can also use these masks individually at any time.

Before applying any facial mask, gently cleanse your skin. Use the refreshing Citrus Splash as an easy, natural way to begin the process.

1. Fill a bowl or the basin with warm water.

2. Squeeze the juice of $^1/_2$ a lemon, lime, or orange into the water.

3. Splash your face with the citrus water—a gentle astringent and a natural antimicrobial agent.

4. Press & Release over the face and neck to stimulate lymph and blood flow in preparation for the maximum absorption of a nutritional mask.

5. Use the Press & Release with a fluffy towel to dry your face and neck.

DEEP NOURISHMENT

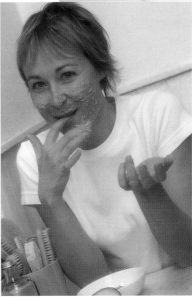

Avocado, often treated and eaten like a vegetable is, in fact, a fruit—the most oil-rich fruit on the planet. It is loaded with goodness. It is a natural moisturizer and rich emollient on its own or as the base for other healing fruits or vegetables. The best part is the green pulp next to the skin. A thin layer of this green pulp can be used under makeup to protect the skin from pollution and grime. Its lubrication can last for hours, and prolonged use can improve the texture of your skin.

1. Slice a fresh avocado in half. Remove the pit and the yellowish portion of the fruit. (You can make guacamole from this unused portion!)

2. Scoop the green pulp into a bowl.

3. Mash the pulp with a fork.

4. Apply to the face and neck using the Sweep & Smooth technique.

5. If you have time, use the Finger Ripple to apply the avocado directly to your closed eyelids, and rest for 20 minutes.

6. Remove the avocado with tepid water, using a loose Press & Release.

Additions

- Add 1 teaspoon of organic oil—coconut, almond, or flax.
- Add 1 teaspoon of organic honey.
- Add equal parts of mashed papaya. The papain in the fruit is a lively rejuvenating enzyme that aids exfoliation.
- Add $1/8$ teaspoon of powdered ginger to the avocado-papaya mask to stimulate circulation. CAUTION: Do not put this mixture on the eyelids!

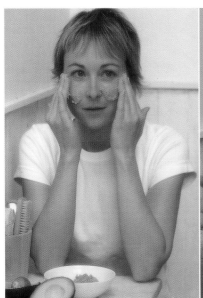
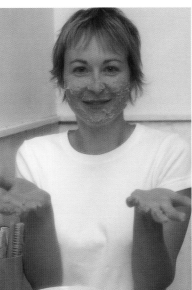

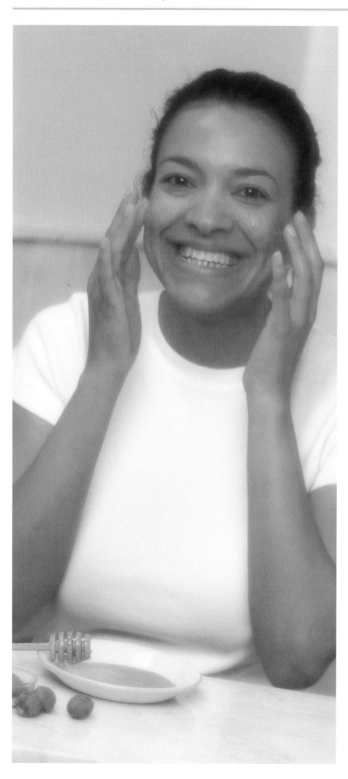

Honey (Royal Nectar)

Honey, a truly royal nectar and the common ingredient in these three masks, is the perfect food created by bees to feed the hive and their queen. The treasure of honey is not in its delectable sweetness but in its profound healing benefits that hydrate, nourish, and tighten the skin. As a natural humectant, honey hydrates by drawing moisture to the skin. Being slightly acidic, it replenishes and protects the skin's acid mantle, healing microabrasions from environmental pollutants and the harsh chemicals found in some skin care products. The enzyme-rich water content aids the healing of blemishes and blackheads.

Nutmeg

Traditionally a holiday spice, it is also a potent natural healer for the skin. Its gentle exfoliating action pulls out impurities on both physical and psychic levels. The honey and nutmeg mixture removes dead skin cells, cleans and refines pores, relieves scarring, and tightens small lines. Exfoliation with this mask is so complete and gentle that your skin will feel as silky as a baby's bottom.

Cream

The wealth of milk is found in its fat-rich cream, which is loaded with enzymes. These enzymes digest the dead outer skin cells. Cream acts as an emollient—it nourishes dry skin, softens wind-burned skin, regenerates sun-baked skin, and rejuvenates debilitated skin.

Eggs

Eggs, whole fertile or free-range, are a nearly perfect food. The balanced blend of lecithin and cholesterol, protein and fat, minerals and vitamins make a whole egg the prime source of nutrients to aid regeneration of skin cells. As a natural astringent, eggs help refine pores while offering nourishment to the skin.

Honey and Nutmeg

The honey tap stimulates lymph and blood circulation, frees holding patterns in the micromuscles, and lifts emotional crystallizations from entrenched positions. This tap is a bone-to-bone connection and a wake-up stimulation to release tension at the densest level. As the bones connect, muscles and facial features relax and skin cells ease into balanced function.

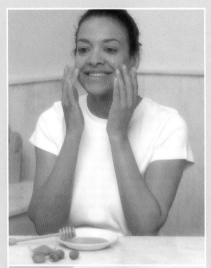

1. Combine $1/2$–1 teaspoon of nutmeg (fresh ground or powdered) with 1 tablespoon of organic honey. (NOTE: Add less fresh nutmeg than powdered as the newly released oils are more potent and may feel warm on delicate skin as circulation is increased.)

2. Use the Finger Ripple to apply the mixture sparingly on your face and neck (too much and your body's heat will melt the honey, causing it to drip!).

3. Honey tap—use your fingertips to tap everywhere on the face, in rapid succession. As your fingers ripple and tap, remember cellular communication. Talk to your cells, "You can release all metabolic wastes; you can receive this nutrition; you can let go of the tightness I do not even feel."

4. Take a moment to focus on your eyelids with an extra-gentle Finger Ripple.

5. Wash your hands, and leave this mask on for 20 minutes.

6. Splash handfuls of warm water over your entire face and neck to loosen and remove the mask.

7. Pat the skin dry, using a gentle Press & Release.

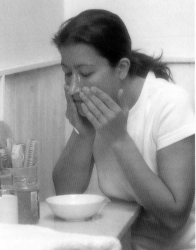

Cream and Honey

1. Add a little more than 1 tablespoon of organic heavy whipping cream to 1 tablespoon of organic honey.

2. Mix with a fork until frothy.

3. Apply the mixture to your face and neck using the Sweep & Smooth.

4. Activate the skin with the Finger Ripple.

5. Reapply the mixture as the skin absorbs it (every 3–5 minutes).

6. Leave on for the magic 20-minute minimum.

7. Use warm water in free-form sweeps to remove this mask.

8. Pat the skin dry, using a gentle Press & Release.

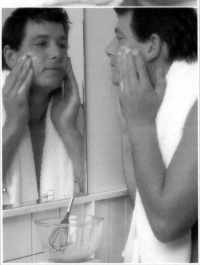

Egg and Honey

1. Beat the whole egg (yolk and white) until it is rich and frothy.

2. Add $1/4$ teaspoon of organic honey and beat again.

3. Apply with the Sweep & Smooth technique along the Rejuv pathways.

4. Leave the mask on for 20 minutes or until the egg sets.

5. Cool-water splashes and free-form sweeps are best to remove this mask.

6. Pat the skin dry, using a gentle Press & Release.

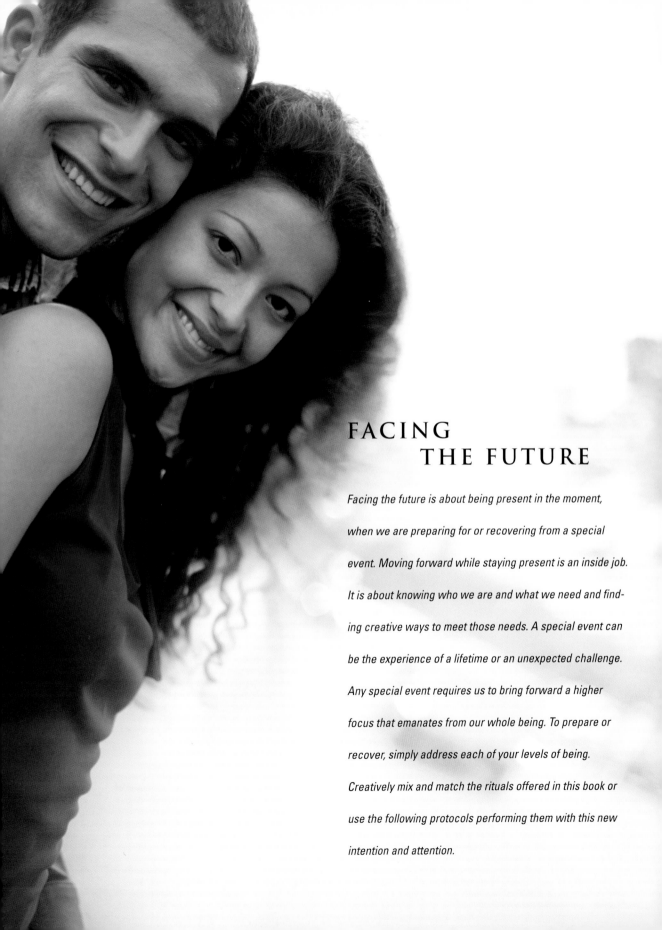

FACING
THE FUTURE

Facing the future is about being present in the moment,

when we are preparing for or recovering from a special

event. Moving forward while staying present is an inside job.

It is about knowing who we are and what we need and find-

ing creative ways to meet those needs. A special event can

be the experience of a lifetime or an unexpected challenge.

Any special event requires us to bring forward a higher

focus that emanates from our whole being. To prepare or

recover, simply address each of your levels of being.

Creatively mix and match the rituals offered in this book or

use the following protocols performing them with this new

intention and attention.

Although preparing ourselves for a special event on all levels may seem like a huge task, it does not have to take a long time; 30–45 minutes is enough. We can rest the body, calm the mind, and balance our emotions during the time it takes to feed our face with a mask. To complete the inner preparation, relax your chakras. We have learned to relax muscles and even organs but seldom have we relaxed chakras—feel them let go and rest.

Mask/Prone Meditation
Inner Preparation

1. Prepare a space to elevate your legs above your heart—in bed with lots of pillows, lying on a slant board, or on the floor with your feet up on a chair.
2. Prepare a honey and nutmeg mask (see page 107) with cool cucumber slices, or warm, wet, black tea bags for your eyes.

Physical Preparation

1. Apply the honey and nutmeg mask. The honey tap exfoliates, giving you a rosy glow.
2. Place slices of cool cucumbers or warm, wet, black tea bags onto your eyelids to reduce puffiness and swelling.
3. Rest your with legs elevated for 20 minutes while gravity works to bring more blood to the brain, refreshing and clearing your mind.

Emotional and Mental Preparation

While you rest, perform the following meditation to release expectations about the upcoming event. Both positive and negative expectations can set you up for disappointment. Expectations take you out of the moment and limit the outcome of any situation.

1. Breathe gently, noticing your thoughts and emotions.
2. Become aware of any expectations you have about the upcoming event: apprehension, anxiety, desire, needs, confusion.
3. One by one, exhale them completely.
4. See, feel, or imagine each expectation dissolving as you exhale.
5. As this process becomes complete, notice that you have created the space for new and unexpected possibilities.

Energetic and Spiritual Preparation

1. Continue with the same gentle breath and focus on your chakras.
2. Bring your awareness to your heart—the fourth chakra—and feel yourself letting go. Relax your heart just as you would a tight muscle. Feel a deep, soft resting place in this chakra. Shift your awareness to your solar plexus—the third chakra—and let go, relax, soften, and rest. Move to the lower abdomen—the second chakra—let go, relax, soften, and rest. Move to the base (root) chakra—the first—and let go, relax, soften, and rest.
3. Return to the heart chakra, relax more deeply, and begin moving your awareness upward. Move to your throat—the fifth chakra—and let go, relax, soften, and rest. Move up to the third eye—the sixth chakra—and repeat. Then shift to the crown—the seventh chakra—and finally to the soul's potential—the eighth chakra.
4. Return to the heart, settle into a resting place, and feel the ease of the whole chakra system. Let your chakras fill with life force. Receive, accept, and absorb the life force as your gift of preparation. Take a few deep, refreshing breaths. Perform the morning stretch, and get up slowly. Take a moment to feel the inner balance of stillness and vitality before removing the mask.
5. Notice the radiance of your face and eyes, the clarity of your mind and emotions. You are now prepared to face this special event with your entire self fully present.

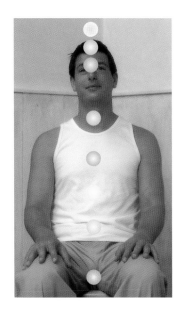

THE CHAKRAS

8. Soul potential

7. Crown

6. Third eye

5. Throat

4. Heart

3. Solar plexus

2. Sacral

1. Root (base)

Supporting your body will enhance the mental and emotional recovery process.
Once your body's chemistry returns to balance, it can lend its molecular,
biochemical support to help you regain peace of mind and emotional stability.
Use this simple regimen for one to three days to recover and renew from stressful
events and circumstances of life.

Physical and Energetic Recovery

Use the elixir of life ritual (see Chapter 5) to energize the water as you increase your
daily intake to 10–12 glasses. Let the water dissolve and eliminate the molecules of
stress from your body, mind, and spirit.

Begin each day with a lemon jump start (see Chapter 5) to alkalinize any acidic
overload in your digestive system.

Add two glasses of Honi-Vin (see Chapter 2) to your fluid intake throughout
each day. Its high mineral and enzyme content will help balance your pH and
replenish critical nutritional needs.

Before your morning shower, dry brush your entire body with a vegetable
bristle body brush (see Chapter 2). Stimulating the nerves all over your skin will
help your adrenal glands to release toxic stress as well as offset energetic overload
and resume balanced function.

Take a brisk 20-minute walk using the shower of light and color (see Chapter 5)
as your visual and mental focus. Let the color flows of cleansing actively refresh
you energetically as you move blood, lymph, muscle, and bone. Your physical and
energetic regenerative systems will synchronize and work together to bring you
into balance.

End each day with a muscle tension buster bath (see Chapter 6) to sweat out
impurities and rebuild the integrity of your electromagnetic field.

Emotional and Mental Recovery

Use the Seven-Count Coupler Pull (see Chapter 5) to balance your emotions as often
as necessary throughout each day.

To relieve emotional and mental overload, use the Rejuv Touch application
ritual (see Chapter 4) without product and with an exceptionally light touch. Your
full presence will penetrate deep into the musculature and bones dissolve emotional
crystallizations and mental holding patterns. As the toxic stress moves through Rejuv
pathways to a nerve center, it can be dissipated or reintegrated. As you Lift to Smile,
let it all go and let the smile lift you—body, mind, and spirit.

Using the deep cleanse (see Chapter 5) to relax your vital energy will help you
release emotional and mental debris from your chakra system. As you cleanse these
energy organs, your physical organ systems also release metabolic wastes and are
restored to balanced function.

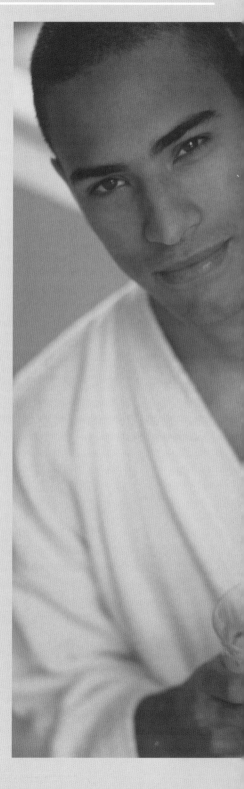

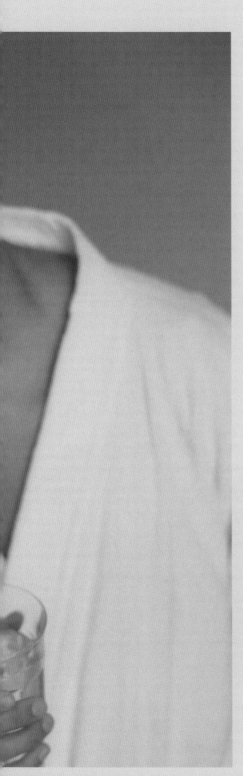

Spiritual Recovery

When we talk about the heart of the matter, we mean the central core of an issue. As the central core of the body, the physical heart is profoundly affected not only by daily physical activities but also by emotional and mental stress patterns. Recovering our own equilibrium is essential; detoxing the overload physically and energetically is a priority. Recovery is a deep multilevel assimilation of the event that lets us truly reap the fruits of our experience and absorb their goodness into body, mind, and spirit.

When we need to recover from an event or situation, the heart in particular requires special care. The healthy functioning of our heart on every level is connected to the quality of our breath. Since the heart rests on the diaphragm, it is directly affected by our breathing. Therefore, controlled breathing is a natural exercise that supports healthy heart functioning. The body is designed so that exercise plays an important role in circulation. As we breathe muscular contractions move the blood and lymph through the body. Healthy circulation of energy from the heart feeds both the physical and spiritual flows within us.

Heart Breath

Using this rhythmic breathing exercise at any time will provide centering and mental clarity. It will also help regulate the heartbeat by slowing the beat and allowing the heart to rest. At rest between beats, the oxygen-rich blood will feed the heart muscle itself.

You can practice the heart breath using different counts as you inhale/exhale. When using any of the methods below, breathe in sets of three. Diaphragmatic breathing to a count of seven is soothing to the heart. Method # 1 is designed to strengthen your diaphragm. To increase your oxygen uptake, method # 2 adds a short hold into the breathing pattern. Build your capacity to breathe rhythmically until the seven counts in each inhale, exhale, and hold are measured by your own heartbeat. Method # 3 provides the deepest rest and support for the heart.

Method # 1:
Breathe in to the count of seven; breathe out to the count of seven.

Method # 2:
Breathe in to the count of seven, hold to the count of two, breathe out to the count of seven, hold to the count of two again.

Method # 3:
Breathe in to the count of seven, hold to the count of seven, breathe out to the count of seven, hold for seven seconds.

7. EASING THE LINES OF LIFE

THE LINES OF EXPRESSION ON OUR FACES ARE THE VISIBLE MAP OF OUR EXPERIENCE—OUR JOYS, OUR SORROWS, OUR STRENGTHS. THESE LINES OF LIFE NEED TO BE EASED AND REFRESHED WITH LOVING ACCEPTANCE, NOT ERASED. THEY TELL THE FULLNESS OF OUR STORIES.

The Daily Rejuv Touch Ritual is the foundation of the advanced protocols in this chapter as we further refine the Pathways of Radiance. We will approach most areas of the face using two methods—first a precise protocol, then Rejuv WrinklEase. Bear in mind that this level of work affects not only the structures of the face but also specific components of the physiological and energetic organ systems as well as the synchronization and communication between them. In HeadWise reflexology (see Chapter 3), the bones, muscles, and contact points are used to reflex the whole system. Once again, we are touching with full presence (not pressure). Increased proficiency of the Rejuv Touch will take these simple sweeps to the next level of healing.

You can create a wrinkle in clothing by bunching the material together: the wrinkle is the gap between the folds, where you cannot see the material. On a cellular level, when a micromuscle contracts, the skin reflexively bunches. Wrinkles are the crevices of tissue you cannot see because the skin is folded. The cells in the crevices are undernourished and dehydrated, hampered in their ability to regenerate by the contracted micromuscles. Some wrinkles are superficial and transient; other crevices are deep and abiding. Bringing your presence, loving intentionality, and cellular communication to the atoms, molecules, cells, and tissues of the wrinkle will enliven the area, your face, and your entire body while opening a space for a deep quality of spiritual renewal to enter. WrinklEase is the Rejuv approach to lightening our perception of wrinkles. With a featherlight touch, the Rejuv WrinklEase protocol loosens and dissolves the emotional crystallizations that have caused the micromuscle contractions. These moments of self-nurturing are designed to ease the stress within the wrinkles, not to remove the lines of expression.

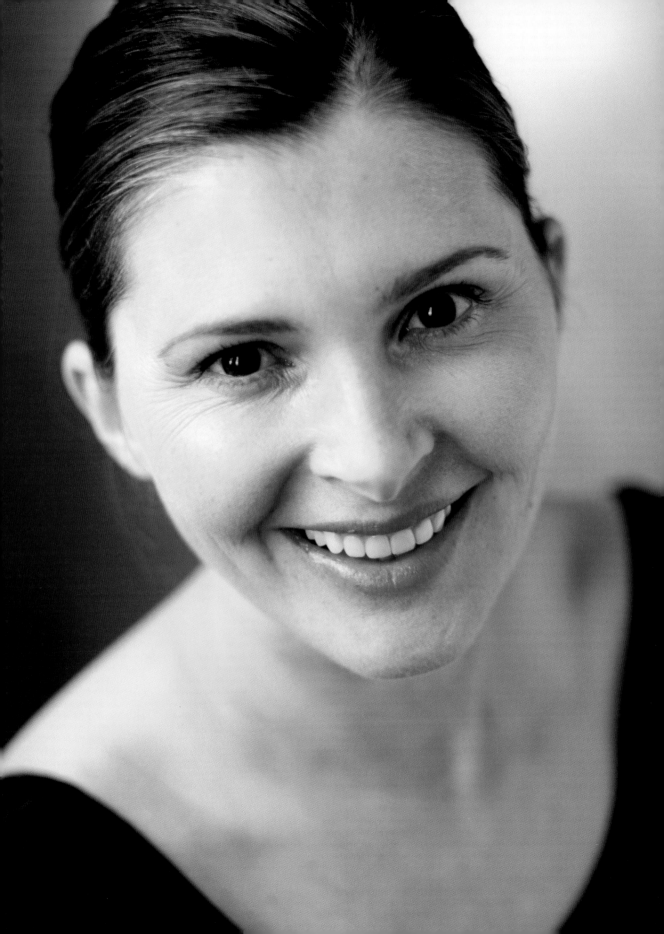

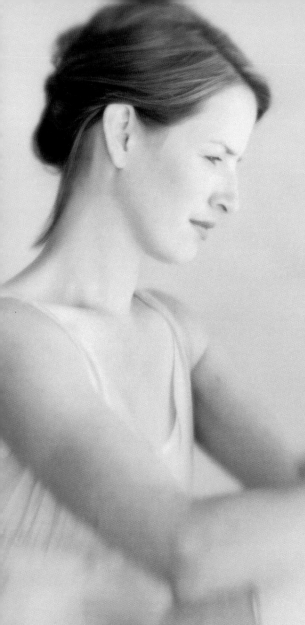

REJUV WRINKLEASE

Regardless of the area affected, the deepest part of a wrinkle is always toward the center of the face. Begin tracing where the wrinkle is deepest and sweep outward as it diminishes. Maintain your awareness on opening and expanding. WrinklEase is done featherlightly on the skin and repeated in the energy field above the skin. Trace the line of the wrinkle beyond its end and into the energy field to provide an energetic direction for dissipation. Moving into the energy field will create a flow for the continual drainage of the emotional crystallizations. Once the energy is released, micromuscles can begin to relax and reshape. Performing WrinklEase often will stabilize the pattern for all the tissues in the area—bone, muscle, blood, lymph, nerve, and skin—to return to their natural state.

THE FOREHEAD

Physically, the forehead is the broad expanse of the frontal bone that protects the brain. Mentally and emotionally, the forehead displays how we think. It holds the effects of our lines of thoughts. The Three-Channel Sweep & Smooth is a deeper refinement of the forehead pathway. Focusing on each channel helps to clear old thought patterns and the excessive mental agitation and brings clarity to the third eye. Your touch is the Rejuv Touch—present, slow, loving, and communicating as you sweep the three arching channels on the forehead (see Chapter 3).

Forehead—Three-Channel Sweep & Smooth

1. Use your middle fingertips and pads sweeping in three channels. Always begin the sweep at the midline between the brows.

Follow the contour of the bone and end at the temples.

2. First channel: Using the middle finger pads, sweep just above the brows, directly to the temples. Hold for three counts, Lift to Smile, hold for another count of three.

3. Second channel: Using the middle finger pads, sweep up the midline to the center of the forehead, open wide across to the temples. Hold for three counts, Lift to Smile, hold for another count of three.

4. Third channel: Using the middle finger pads, sweep up the midline to just below the hairline, following the arch to the temples. Hold for three counts, Lift to Smile, hold for another count of three.

5. To end, touch the pituitary point, then touch the crown point (see page 75, # 6 a–c).

WRINKLEASE FOR THE FOREHEAD

The lines of expression on our forehead can deepen into major wrinkles. These wrinkles can be horizontal, vertical (between the brows), on the left, on the right, or across the midline and extending to both sides. The same micromuscles that contract a hundred times a day over this broad expanse of bone, muscle, and skin can be eased with this specific WrinklEase technique.

If a horizontal wrinkle crosses the midline, use both hands. Simultaneously placing two fingertips at the center of the wrinkle, trace outward to both ends of the wrinkle, then into the energy field. If a wrinkle is vertical, the deepest point will be closer to the nose. Place your fingertip at this point and trace up the wrinkle toward the hairline, lifting into the energy field 3–5 inches (8–12 cm) as the physical wrinkle ends. If the wrinkle is diagonal, crooked, or broken, just follow its direction as best you can from the deepest point to the least visible on the skin, then out into the energy field.

First—On the Skin

Trace with a touch that is light but makes a bone-to-bone connection.

1. Place your fingertip at the deepest point of the wrinkle.

2. Trace outward with a featherlight touch to the point where the physical wrinkle disappears on the skin (the least visible part of the wrinkle).

3. Continue tracing the line off the face into the energy field as though

it were a continuation of the physical wrinkle. See, feel, or imagine a string of energy flowing out with your fingertip.

4. Pull the string of energy out beyond the end of the physical wrinkle into the energy field, 3–5 inches (8–12 cm) until you sense it end and dissolve.

5. Trace this wrinkle outward three times before moving to another one.

Second—In the Energy Field

6. Follow the same placement and procedure as on the skin but do the tracing in the energy field, 2 inches (5 cm) above the skin.

7. Trace outward to the end of the wrinkle and continue.

8. Pull the string of energy out beyond the end of the wrinkle farther into the energy field 6–8 inches (15–20 cm), until you sense it dissolve.

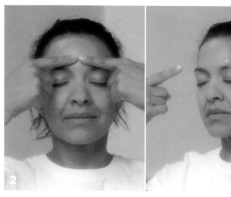

Our eyes continuously process the visual input of our daily lives. We look out at our world and our world flows right back in, loaded with light, color, texture, and shape. This advanced Rejuv protocol rests, energizes, and strengthens your eyes as it refines the pathway.

You begin and end this ritual the same way, by cupping your palm chakras over the eyes. Use the Finger Ripple around the orbital ridge of the upper and lower eyes to enliven and stimulate the full-body reflex points located around the eyes.

Palm the Eyes to Relax

1. Rub hands together to energize the palm chakras and warm the skin.

2. Cup your palms and cover your eyes, aligning your palm chakras directly over your eyeballs. If you blink your eyes, you should barely feel your lashes brushing your palms.

3. Adjust your palms so the eyes receive little or no light.

4. Hold, resting in the warmth of your touch. (You can place your elbows onto a table or rest your arms on your chest so the hold can be comfortably sustained.)

5. Communicate, sending your loving intention into all the tissues— the lids, all the eye structures, the optic nerve, and the brain.

6. Release your hands from your eyes; open them slowly.

Upper-Eye Finger Ripple

7. Place your ring finger tip near the bridge of the nose, middle, and index finger pads along the brows on the edge of the upper orbital bone.

8. Your fingers will be slightly curved, tips touching the brow hair.

9. In a slow, steady ripple, ring-press, middle-press, index-press, move in tiny increments to the outer corner of the eye.

10. When the index finger reaches the outer corner, use it to trace up and out to the temple points.

11. Hold for a count of three, Lift to Smile, hold for another count of three.

12. Repeat three times.

13. To end, touch the pituitary point, then touch the crown point (see page 75, # 6a–c).

Lower-Eye Finger Ripple

14. Begin by placing your ring fingertip near the bridge of the nose, middle, and index fingertips along the lower orbital ridge.

15. Your fingers will be slightly curved, nails touching the lashes of the lower lids. (With very long nails, use the pads of the fingers.)

16. In a slow, steady ripple, ring-press, middle-press, index-press, move in tiny increments to the outer corner of the eye.

17. Repeat steps # 10–13, as above.

18. Palm the eyes to complete this ritual.

PALM THE EYES   UPPER EYE

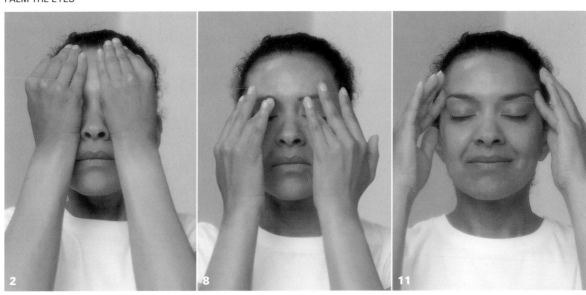

2   8   11

We approach the eyes with delicacy, reverence, and an even lighter touch. To maximize the expansion and lift, focus your positive attention on each eye individually. First trace the lines on the lid, from inner to outer corner, then the lines radiating out from the outer corner of the eyes. Trace these tiny lines with a featherlight touch that is barely physical yet makes a penetrating connection.

First—On the Skin

1. Place your middle fingertip at the deepest point of the wrinkle, following its direction, near the corner of the eye where a line begins.

2. Trace outward with a featherlight touch; stay in contact with the skin for only the length of the wrinkle, following its direction.

3. Continue tracing the line off the face into the energy field as though it were a continuation of the physical wrinkle. See, feel, or imagine a string of energy flowing out with your fingertip.

4. Pull the string of energy out beyond the end of the physical wrinkle into the energy field 3–5 inches (8–12 cm).

5. Trace this wrinkle three times before moving to another wrinkle.

6. Repeat on the other eye.

Second—In the Energy Field

7. Follow the same placement and procedure as on the skin, but do the tracing in the energy field, 2 inches (5 cm) above the skin of the eye.

8. Trace each tiny line from its deepest point to its lightest and on into the energy field.

9. Pull the string of energy beyond the end of the wrinkle farther into the energy field 6–8 inches (15–20 cm) until you sense it dissolve.

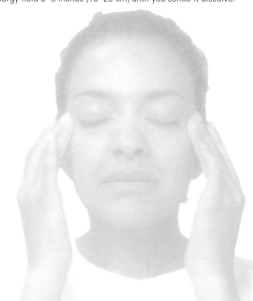

LOWER EYE (ON THE SKIN)

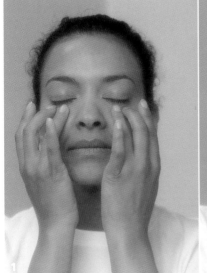
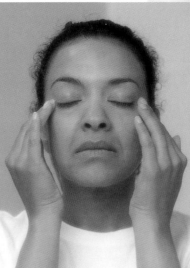
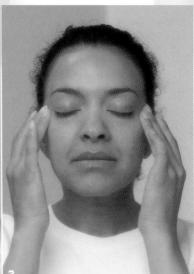

The nose brings us that enchanting whiff of jasmine, the tang of an ocean breeze, the aroma of fresh-baked bread. Yet the nose rarely receives much attention unless it begins to run, sneeze, or tickle. We seldom acknowledge that the breath of life with its oxygen, prana, and all the richness of life's scents enters through the nose, where that air is filtered and moistened, where prana is guided to the brain, where scents are absorbed.

The Bridge Sweep relaxes the tissue and cartilage of the nose, integrating its whole structure with the broad expanse of the forehead and connecting breath with the third eye. You will bring your awareness to the nerves within the entrance for your breath as it opens and eases the intake of air and prana.

The Nostril Flair Sweep releases tension and tightness held in the delicate flair of the nostrils and allows them to soften and open. This flair of tissue is responsive to many emotions that play through our beings. As the nostrils relax, their ease radiates into the cheeks and lips, and the whole face softens.

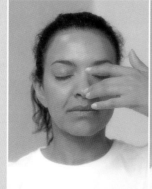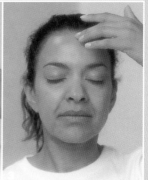
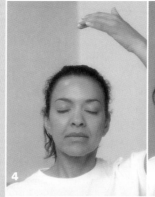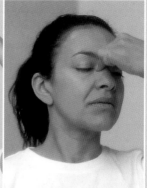
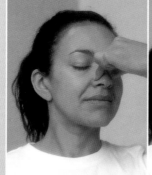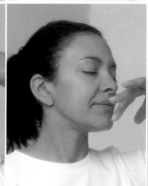

Bridge Sweep

This is a spreadable stroke. Imagine that you are spreading thick, rich honey along the midline of the face from the tip of the nose to the hairline. The sweep is gentle and slow.

1. Place the pad of one middle finger at the tip of your nose.

2. Sweep your finger pad upward on the flat of the bridge of the nose. Feel the hills and hollows beneath your finger pad as you sweep.

3. Dip into the hollow where the nose meets the forehead and continue sweeping vertically up the midline of the forehead, over the third eye area, to the hairline.

4. Release your touch upward into the energy field toward the eighth chakra.

5. Repeat the sweep three, six, or nine times, as feels appropriate.

6. To end, touch the pituitary point, then touch the crown point.

Nostril Flair Sweep

Your finger pads stroke softly and loosely throughout the sweep.

7. Place the thumb and index finger pad of one hand at the sides of the bridge of the nose near the eyes.

8. Simultaneously sweep thumb and finger pad down, following the contours of the sides of the nose and the flair of the nostrils. Fingertips pass the nose points and continue into the energy field below the nose.

9. As you leave the flair of the nostrils and continue in the energy field, open the space between thumb and finger, creating a bell shape. This reinforces the openness of the energetic structures of the nostrils. Remind your nose to remain open as you softly breathe.

10. Repeat the sweep three, six, or nine times, as feels appropriate.

11. To end, touch the pituitary point, then touch the crown point (see page 75, # 6 a–c).

THE CHEEKS

Cheekbones are a prominent feature and give breadth, definition, and shape to our faces. The Three-Channel Sweep & Smooth offers a deep activation of the Rejuv pathway within the bones and muscles of the cheek area. The spongy cheek tissue is a reflex point for the lungs. This sweep brings integration to the entire breathing system from nose to lungs. Sweep across the wide expanse of the cheekbones, opening toward the coronal plane, and gently assisting the musculature as it lifts. Do not follow the downward shape of the lower cheekbone, as this will cause the cheek tissue to sag rather than to lift.

Cheeks—Three-Channel Sweep & Smooth

Middle finger pads will sweep in three channels beginning at the midline of the nose, at the top of each channel. With each sweep, slide gently down the sides of the nose and into the Rejuv pathway on the cheeks, then open widely to the designated nerve center.

1. First channel: Place your middle finger pads onto the tip of the nose, sweep down the sides of the nose following the contours of the flair of the nostrils to the nose points, hold for three counts, Lift to Smile, hold for another count of three. Continue the sweep across the tread of the lower cheekbone to the triangle ear points, hold for three counts, Lift to Smile, hold for another count of three.

2. Second channel: Place your middle finger pads on the middle of the nose at the midline, sweep down the nose and across the flat of the cheekbone to the triangle ear points, hold for three counts, Lift to Smile, hold for another count of three.

3. Third channel: Place your middle finger pads onto the midline at the bridge of the nose near the inner corner of the eyes, sweep down the nose around the lower eye to the temples. Hold for a three counts, Lift to Smile, and hold for another count of three.

4. To end, touch the pituitary point, then touch the crown point (see page 75, # 6 a–c).

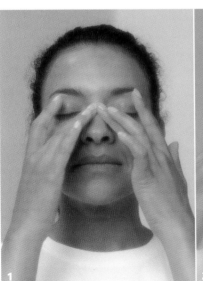
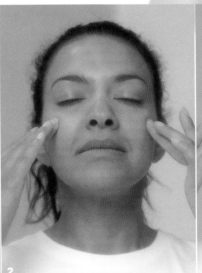
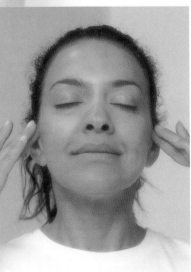

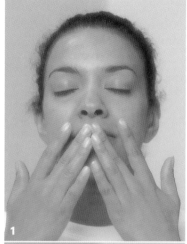

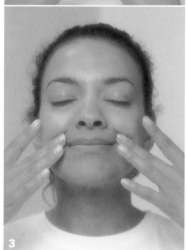

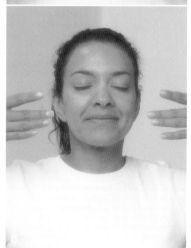

The mouth and lips appear to be comprised of a single expressive muscle. Actually they are a cluster of muscles working in concert as we eat, talk, grimace, or laugh. We approach the mouth with full presence and virtually no pressure. Loving delicacy is the key. The cosmic grin is a gentle reminder to smile from the heart. With this gentle touch, the musculature relaxes, free to flash the world a genuine, spontaneous grin. This technique is about remembering to be tender and compassionate with ourselves, both about the things we said and wish we had not, and the things we wish we had said but did not.

Cosmic Grin to Cheshire Grin

1. Place your middle finger pads at the midline, touching both your upper and lower lips.

2. Sweep with a featherlight touch to the mouth corner points. Hold for a count of three.

3. Lift to Smile, fingertips delicately lifting the mouth corners at a 45-degree angle, with as little distortion of the musculature of the mouth as possible. Hold for a count of three.

4. Your middle fingertips stay in the lift at the mouth corner points as your elbows lift to the sides and you place your thumbs at the parotid points. Hold both for a count of three.

5. Gently Lift to Smile, using both middle fingers and thumbs, hold for a count of three.

6. Remain in this position as you imagine a smile that starts at your lips, opens across your lower cheeks to the parotid points, flows out along your forearms to your elbows, and pours outward into your energy field into a cosmic grin.

7. Lift to Smile, in a 45-degree angle, at parotid and mouth corner points, hold for a count of three.

8. Release your fingers and thumbs from the nerve centers, and slowly draw them outward in the same 45-degree angle of smile, pulling the cosmic grin into a Cheshire grin in your energy field.

9. Stop just beyond your ears, bringing middle fingertip and thumb together; hold the wide Cheshire grin.

10. As you hold the Cheshire grin, think of something that you absolutely adore, that gives you delight and joy, that makes you smile inside. Feel that delight like a bubble in your belly. Enjoy the delight, and let it grow bigger and bigger within you.

11. Radiate that delight through the Cheshire grin. Let it continue to stream outward and upward toward the far corners of the universe into an even bigger cosmic grin. Feel the lift and expansion on all levels of your being.

12. To end, release fingers and thumbs, and use both middle fingers to touch first the pituitary point and then the crown point (see page 75, # 6 a–c).

WRINKLEASE FOR THE MOUTH AND LIPS

Our lips are almost constantly in motion and play a leading role in our moment-to-moment communication. As we age, tiny little lines appear around our lips and radiate out into the surrounding skin in a sunburst pattern. The WrinklEase technique will open and soften these tiny lines and wrinkles around the lips.

The Sunburst for Lips

To ground and stabilize your hands for this delicate work, put the edges of your hands and sides of your wrists together, palms almost facing you. Lean the edges into each other. Feel their stability. Then rest your upper arms against your chest. Now your middle finger pads are supported and free to do WrinklEase for the lips.

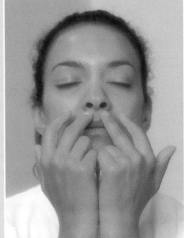

First—On the Skin

Use a flicking motion (a tiny tracing) with a touch that is light but has a penetrating connection.

1. At the midline, place your middle fingertips at the edge of the rose color of your upper lip, touching both lip and skin tissue.

2. Flick the tips of the middle fingers away from the lips with a featherlight touch. The fingertip may move only a fraction of an inch or longer, but you should stay in contact with the skin only for the length of the wrinkle.

3. See, feel, or imagine a tiny string of energy flicking off with the motion of your fingertip.

4. Pull the string of energy just a little farther beyond the end of the lip tissue until you sense it end and dissolve.

5. Flick your fingertip out over this wrinkle three times before moving your finger out toward the mouth corner points.

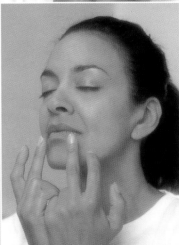

6. Repeat the flick all along the edge of the upper lips until you reach the mouth corner points. Hold for a count of three, Lift to Smile, and hold for another count of three.

7. Repeat the same process on the lower lip.

Second—In the Energy Field

8. Follow the same placement and procedure as above but do the whole sunburst in the energy field, 2 inches (5 cm) above the upper and lower lips, holding and lifting to smile at the mouth corner points.

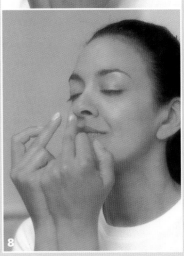

The neck is more than a column to adorn with jewels, high collars, or scarves. The neck is miraculously engineered to support a 10–12 pound (4.5–5.5 kg) head. It keeps the head upright against the force of gravity and permits turning, bending, and arching with grace and fluidity.

This simple sweep on the neck begins to clear the crystallizations stored in and around physical structures critical to our survival: our trachea so we can breathe, our esophagus so we can eat and drink, our spinal cord so we can move. The skin, tissue, and muscles of the neck are lifted and supported to resist gravity's pull.

The Neck Fan

Sweep with both the right and left hands simultaneously. Use the flat of your index finger and the middle finger knuckles of both hands. Each pass begins at the hollow, sweeps up to the riser of the jawbone, and releases into the energy field.

1. Place the flats of your knuckles into the hollow.

2. Both hands smoothly sweep up the midline of the neck to the riser of the jawbone and release into the energy field.

3. Return your knuckles to the hollow.

4. Sweep from the hollow to the middle of the jawbone and release into the energy field.

5. Return your knuckles to the hollow.

6. Sweep from the hollow to the parotid points. Hold with the knuckle tip for a count of three.

7. Remain in place and elegantly slide from knuckle to fingertip at the parotid points. Lift to Smile, and hold for a count of three.

8 a–b. Begin to slide the length of your finger up the sides of the head until your full hand is in contact and sliding up the coronal plane.

9. Continue the slide until your middle fingers touch the crown point. Hold the crown for a count of three.

10. Release your fingers and hands upward toward the eighth chakra. Feel the flow of the lift.

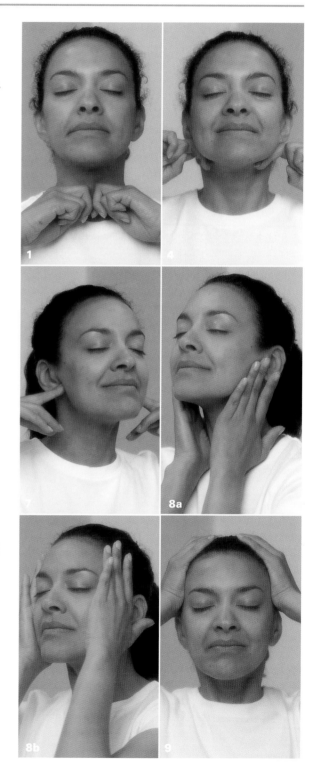

WRINKLEASE FOR THE NECK

Along with all the physical structures for survival, the neck also houses the larynx, the thyroid and parathyroid glands, and the throat chakra. We use WrinklEase with delicacy and tenderness in the touch not only to ease the lines on the neck but also to release the weight of the crystallizations locked within these structures.

First—On the Skin

Trace with a touch that is light but makes a penetrating connection.

1. Place both your middle fingertips at the center of a wrinkle on the neck.

2. Simultaneously trace the line of a horizontal wrinkle out toward the coronal plane with a featherlight touch, staying in contact with the skin for only the length of the wrinkle.

3. Continue tracing the line off the neck into the energy field to both sides as though it were a continuation of the physical wrinkle. See, feel, or imagine a string of energy flowing out with your fingertips.

4. Pull the string of energy beyond the end of the physical wrinkle into the energy field 3–5 inches (8–12 cm) until you sense it end and dissolve.

5. Trace this wrinkle outward three times before moving to another wrinkle. If the wrinkle is diagonal, crooked, or broken, just follow its direction as best you can from the deepest point to the least visible on the skin, then out into the energy field.

Second—In the Energy Field

6. Follow the same placement and procedure as above, but do the tracing in the energy field 2 inches (5 cm) above the skin.

7. Trace outward to the end of the wrinkle and continue.

8. Pull the string of energy beyond the end of the wrinkle even farther into the energy field, 6–8 inches (15–20 cm) until you sense it end and dissolve.

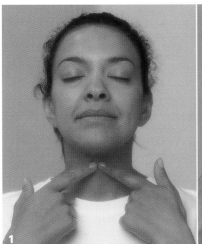

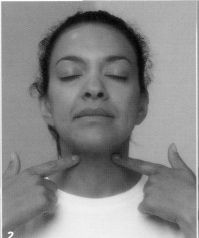

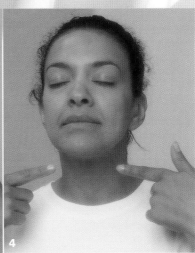

Another powerful reflex area is the jawbone. The tip of the chin (where a cleft is sometimes visible) reflexes the pubic bone, and the temporomandibular joint (TMJ) reflexes the pelvis and hip joints. The pelvis muscles and bones need to be in a relaxed state to maintain equilibrium. As we focus on expanding the chin cleft and strengthening the energetic flow to the nerve centers, we will reflexively open the pubic bone and the hips.

This sweep is a simple and potent way to work both areas and release patterns of contractions simultaneously within the jaw, the pelvic girdle, and the root chakra. We focus on defining and refining a clean chin line—one that is free of sagging skin and drooping jowls.

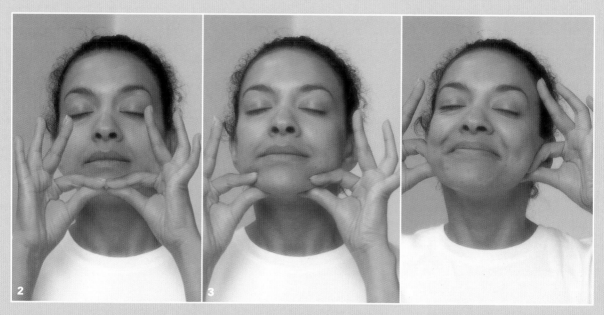

Clean Chin Line Sweep & Smooth

The thumb and index finger sweep together along the length of the jawbone to define a clean chin line.

1. Place your thumb and index finger at the midline—the cleft—of your chin.

2. Your thumb is on the riser and your index finger is on the tread of the jawbone, slightly apart so the edge of the bone peeks through.

3. Begin at the chin cleft and Sweep & Smooth along the jawbone. Sweep slowly enough to feel the nooks and crannies of the bone and any tautness in the muscles.

4. Sweep toward the parotid points.

5. When your fingers reach the ramus of the jaw, join index to thumb and trace both to the parotid points; hold for a count of three.

6. Lift to Smile, and hold for a count of three.

Some signs of aging are inevitable since muscle and connective tissue do lose some of their elasticity over time. However, double and triple chins are the result of poor dietary choices as well as age and gravity. We cannot turn back the clock or stop the pull of gravity, but we can make better nutritional choices, hydrate internally to aid detoxification and regain some of the elasticity that has been lost. By doing the Tuck It Up & In on a daily basis, we can reeducate the muscles and tissues that have responded to the pull of gravity by sagging. The power of the Tuck It Up & In is in the combination of a simple physical process with cellular communication and visualization under your loving touch. As the last ritual for the WrinklEase, be aware of the process you are completing, work with deliberate slowness and receive the fullness of the Rejuv Touch.

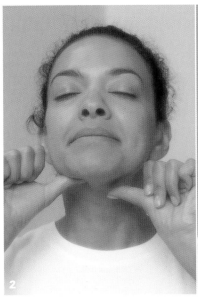
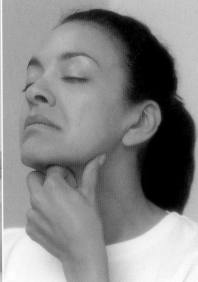
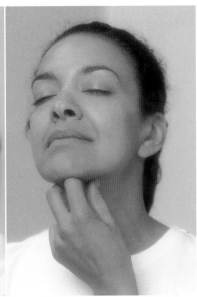

Tuck It Up & In

1. Place the pads of your thumbs in the basket of muscle and connective tissue beneath your chin where extra flesh gathers.

2. Slowly and rhythmically, press your thumbs upward into that basket of soft tissue; use your thumbs to tuck the excess tissue back into the basket where it belongs; tuck tissue from the sides near the underside of the jawbone to the center of the basket. Tuck it up and in.

3. Communicate. Tell the tissue to go back where it belongs. Visualize the tissue redistributing while tone and balance return to the micromuscles. See, feel, or imagine this happening.

4. The final tuck and gather is done with the thumb and fingers of just one hand.

5. Place your thumb and fingers into the center of this basket of tissue under the chin and, as you bring them together, gather all the tissue you can into that center.

6. Do one final press, gently but as deeply as is comfortable, upward toward the crown of the head.

7. Hold for a count of seven while you breathe and draw the energy of your breath upward through the center of your head to the crown and beyond. Communicate. Tell the tissue to reconnect in its perfect physiological alignment.

8. Release the hand that is holding the tissue, and touch the pituitary point, then touch the crown point (see page 75, # 6 a–c).

RECOMMENDED RESOURCES

Education and Training

Burnham Systems Studies provides continuing education, seminars, lectures, and training for professionals, spas and corporations, and the general public in all the concepts presented in the book:

- Physical-Spiritual medicine— philosophy and application.
- The Rejuv Touch, Nerve Centers and Pathways, The Daily Rejuv Touch Ritual and Rejuv Spa Basics.
- WiseBody Therapeutics—a series focusing on the body's full spectrum of "magic buttons" for health—herbs, nutrition, and bodywork that addresses the unique needs of each body system.
- Burnham Systems Facial Rejuvenation: Four-Phase Professional Certification.

For further information and current certified Burnham Systems Facial Rejuvenation practitioners in the United States—call the office or visit the web site.

Office

369 Montezuma Ave. # 346
Santa Fe, NM 87501
(505) 989-1807

Web

www.burnhamsystems.com
burnhamsystems@earthlink.net

Products

Jurlique, regarded as the purest skin care on earth, is grown organically and bio-dynamically, spygerically processed (a specific and time-consuming method of processing herbal products to the highest vibration) in South Australia. Jurlique goes to great lengths to insure the utmost purity and highest quality in all their products. Order through burnhamsystems.com and link to Jurlique or call 800-854-1110.

Dr. Hauschka—organic and bio-dynamic products for the skin:
www.drhauschka.com
800-247-9907

Weleda International—organic and bio-dynamic products for personal care and use:
www.weleda.com
800-265-2615

Aveda—plant-based products for the skin and hair:
www.aveda.com
866-823-1425

Eternal Essence—offers high quality dry-skin brushing kit (three brushes, instructional video, and booklet):
www.info@womenswaves.org
808-335-0959

Reading

Anatomy of the Spirit
Caroline Myss, Ph.D.
Three Rivers Press, 1996

Enzyme Nutrition
Dr. Edward Howell
Avery Publishing, 1985

Esoteric Anatomy
Bruce Burger
North Atlantic Books, 1998

Fats and Oils
Udo Erasmus
Alive Books, 1986

Hands of Light
Barbara Ann Brennan
Bantam Books, 1998

Molecules of Emotions
Candace D. Pert, Ph.D.
Touchstone, 1997

The Chemistry of Man
Dr. Bernard Jensen, Ph.D.
Bernard Jensen Enterprise, 1983

The School of Natural Medicine
Dr. John Christopher
Christopher Publications, 1996

Your Body's Many Cries for Water
F. Batmanghelidj, M.D.
Global Health Solutions, 1992

INDEX

lungs 29
lymphatic system 59, 60, 85, 103

M

meditation 51, 56, 94, 96, 109
mental attitude 13, 14, 20, 78
micromuscles 17, 48, 54, 59, 112, 114
midsagittal plane 40, 46
mind
  calming 38
  recovery rituals 110
  relaxation ritual 95
  special event preparation 109
  two aspects 37
  wake up ritual 82
morning rituals 59, 80–83
mouth 43, 44, 47, 70–71, 120–121
musculature
  easing contractions 7, 17, 112
  enlivening 34, 102, 110
  expression lines 7, 10, 17, 112
  gravity impact 14, 15
  micromuscles 17, 48, 54, 59

N

nerve center points 34, 38, 40, 42, 43
nerve pathways
  cellular communication 17
  function 46–47
  location 40–41, 46–47
  opening 7, 16, 34, 38, 46
  review exercise 58
nose 43, 44, 118
nutmeg 106, 107
nutrition
  detoxification 20, 29, 32
  healing drinks 89
  poor 22, 23, 125
  rejuvenating 24–26
  for skin 104

O

oils
  in diet 24, 25
  in skin 31
organs 20, 28–31, 89

P

papaya 105
parotid points 43, 45
Pathways to Radiance 62
perspiration 31
pituitary point 43–44, 82, 119, 125
pollution 17, 22, 23, 24, 29
presence
  exercises 52, 56, 57, 86
  importance 51, 55, 62
  WrinklEase 112
Press & Release 54, 55, 57, 59, 60, 61
prolapses 14, 16
Psychic Stress Release Bath 101
purification 32–33, 84–87

R

recharging rituals 88–91
recovery rituals 110–111
reflexology 34, 38–39, 86, 112, 124
Rejuvanatomy 40
Rejuv Breath Meditation 51, 56
Rejuv Drop 52
Rejuv Touch system
  benefits 7, 9, 16
  daily rituals 48–75, 112
  healing process 19
  loving intentionality 51–52
  presence 51, 52, 55, 56, 62
Rejuv WrinklEase 112, 114–125
relaxation 17, 18, 92–97, 110
release
  emotional crystallization 17, 18–19, 54
  energy 9, 16, 17, 34, 46, 54
  stress 17, 93, 101, 110
respiratory system 28, 29
riser 41

S

sacred space 52
self
  balancing rituals 83, 90, 110
  inner 7, 9, 10, 33, 78
  nurturing 52, 77, 78
  presence 51, 52, 55, 56, 62, 86
  who are we 13, 38
self-care rituals
  baths 101–103
  daily 78–97
  facial masks 104–107, 109
  recharging 88–91
  relaxation 92–97
  special event preparations 109
  special healing treats 98–111
  wake up and face the day 80–83
  water purification 85–87
skin
  detoxification 28, 30–31, 32–33
  dry skin brushing 32, 110
  facial masks 104–107, 109
  structure 31
sleep, preparation rituals 95, 97
Soak to Save Your Face 60
special event preparations 109
spirit
  inner guidance exercise 33
  nourishing 20, 23, 26
  special event preparation 109
  spiritual body 13, 37
  stressful event recovery 111
stress
  detoxification 25, 33, 110
  release 17, 93, 101, 110
Sweep & Smooth
  Rejuv Touch Ritual 54, 55, 57, 61, 62–75, 110
  WrinklEase 115, 118, 122, 124

T

temple points 43, 45, 82
tension, release 17, 102, 110
touch 52, 53

Touch of Calm ritual 95
toxins
  see also detoxification
  in body 30, 31, 59, 60, 61
  in food 23, 24, 25
  stress release 110
trauma 9, 13, 14, 16, 18–19
tread 41

U

uplifting rituals 55

V

vinegar, cider 33, 101
visualization 82, 85, 94, 95, 110
vitality, enhancing 20, 22, 23, 24

W

water
  baths 98, 101–103
  daily rituals 60, 84–87, 110
  energized 87, 110
  energy source 23, 24, 26, 85
  requirement 23, 25, 32, 88, 110
  within body 29
wrinkles 17, 31, 112–125

PICTURE ACKNOWLEDGMENTS

The Bridgewater Book Company
would like to thank the following
for the permission to reproduce
copyright material: Corbis pp.12
(Rory McNahon), 16 (Claudia Kunin),
32 (Maureen Barrymore),
77 (LWA–Stephen Welstead),
96 (Dennis Degnan), 100 (Jutta Klee),
103 (Jose Luis Pelaez), 104 (Janet
Fish), 114 (Allen Kennedy). Getty
Images (Stone) p.80 (Robert Daley).

Author's cover photograph by
Mateo Galvano.